MAINTENANCE THERAPY
FOR THE GERIATRIC PATIENT

MAINTENANCE THERAPY FOR THE GERIATRIC PATIENT

Compiled and Edited by

JACOB L. RUDD, M.D.

Chief, Physical Medicine and Rehabilitation Service
Veterans Administration Outpatient Clinic
Boston, Massachusetts

and

REUBEN J. MARGOLIN, Ed.D.

Chairman, Department of Rehabilitation and Special Education
Northeastern University
Boston, Massachusetts

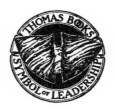

CHARLES C THOMAS • PUBLISHER
Springfield • Illinois • U.S.A.

Published and Distributed Throughout the World by
CHARLES C THOMAS • PUBLISHER
BANNERSTONE HOUSE
301-327 East Lawrence Avenue, Springfield, Illinois, U.S.A.
NATCHEZ PLANTATION HOUSE
735 North Atlantic Boulevard, Fort Lauderdale, Florida, U.S.A.

With THOMAS BOOKS *careful attention is given to all details of
manufacturing and design. It is the Publisher's desire to present books
that are satisfactory as to their physical qualities and artistic possibilities
and appropriate for their particular use.* THOMAS BOOKS *will be true
to those laws of quality that assure a good name and good will.*

Printed in the United States of America
X-2

CONTRIBUTORS

Marie M. Alexander, M.S.
Research Assistant, Department of Nutrition
Harvard University School of Public Health
Boston, Massachusetts

Marvin S. Arffa, Ed.D.
Associate Professor of Social Science
Northeastern University, Boston, Massachusetts
Psychology Consultant
Massachusetts Rehabilitation Commission

Benjamin Bell, M.D.
Chief of Staff and Chief of Normative Aging Study
Veterans Administration Outpatient Clinic
Boston, Massachusetts
Associate Clinical Professor of Otolaryngology
Lecturer in Ophthalmology
Boston University School of Medicine
Boston, Massachusetts

William H. Chasen, M.D.
Chief of the Veterans Administration Arthritis Clinic
Clinical Instructor in Medicine
Boston University School of Medicine
Boston, Massachusetts

George J. Goldin, Ph.D.
Associate Professor of Social Science
Research Director, New England Rehabilitation Institute
Northeastern University, Boston, Massachusetts

William B. Hadley, M.D.
Senior Physician, Joslin Clinic
New England Deaconess Hospital
Boston, Massachusetts

James C. Hunt
Regional Representative, Administration on the Aging
Boston, Massachusetts

v

Reuben J. Margolin, Ed.D.
**Professor of Social Science in Education
Chairman, Department of Rehabilitation and Special Education
Project Director
New England Rehabilitation Research and Demonstration Institute
Northeastern University, Boston, Massachusetts**

Harry T. Phillips, M.D., D.PH.
**Chief of the Bureau of Chronic Disease Control
Massachusetts Department of Public Health
Superintendent, Lemuel Shattuck Hospital, Jamaica Plain, Mass.
Lecturer, Health Services Administration
Harvard University, Cambridge, Massachusetts
Lecturer, Brandeis University, Waltham, Massachusetts and
Tufts University Medical School, Medford, Massachusetts**

Charles L. Rose, A.M.
**Research Coordinator, Normative Aging Study
Veterans Administration Outpatient Clinic
Course Coordinator in Social Work, University College
Northeastern University, Boston, Massachusetts
Project Director, Research Methods Practicum
Boston College School of Social Work
Chestnut Hill, Massachusetts**

Jacob L. Rudd, M.D.
**Chief of the Physical Medicine and Rehabilitation Service
Veterans Administration Outpatient Clinic
Consultant in Rehabilitation Medicine, Boston City Hospital
Consultant to the Department of Rehabilitation
Northeastern University, Boston, Massachusetts
President, North American Academy of Manipulation Medicine**

Frederick J. Stare, Ph.D., M.D.
**Professor of Nutrition
Chairman, Department of Nutrition
Harvard University School of Public Health
Boston, Massachusetts**

Bernard A. Stotsky, Ph.D., M.D.
**Project Director, Study of Mental Patients in Nursing Homes
University Psychiatrist, Northeastern University
Boston, Massachusetts**

This book is dedicated to our wives
Dorothy and Ruth

PREFACE

THIS BOOK was written because we feel that the concept of maintenance therapy should receive increased attention in the treatment of the geriatric patient. The idea of long-term treatment is not original, and we do not make any claims on originality. However, we have attempted to place the concept of maintenance therapy in a new or different frame of reference. It is hoped that this will encourage greater attention to factors which are often overlooked or minimized in treatment.

Every concept has a historical development. Our perception of maintenance therapy emerges from the respective experiences of both editors in related fields which add up to a total of fifty years in rehabilitation. We first became aware of the importance of prolonged therapy when both of us were active in the Physical Medicine and Rehabilitation Service of the Veterans Administration Hospital in Brockton, Massachusetts. At that time we stressed the importance of a modified "total push" program for our geriatric psychiatric patients, many of whom had not only mental but also multiple physical disabilities. Our immediate aim was not to rehabilitate these aged patients back to employment: our goal was to provide them with an activity program in the hospital which would prevent the deconditioning phenomena and help make their lives more meaningful and worthwhile.

The results were surprising though not totally unexpected. Twenty-five per cent of the patients were discharged to their own homes or to foster home care. A few were able to secure employment. A more detailed history of one of the employed patients is presented in Chapter II, "The Role of Physical Medicine and Rehabilitation in Maintenance Therapy." A schizophrenic individual, he secured work in the community, at sixty-five years of age, after twenty years of hospitalization, and was still working at the age of eighty. Many of the other patients in these geriatric wards showed considerable improvement in their physical and psychological conditions. Despite inevitable aging with its accompanying multiple disabilities, they were being maintained in an active state which, for them, was therapeutic.

In November 1959, Jacob L. Rudd was assigned to the Veterans Administration Outpatient Clinic in Boston as Chief of Physical Medicine and Rehabilitation Service. Reuben J. Margolin accepted a professional position with Northeastern University, Boston, Massachusetts, and shortly thereafter was appointed consultant to the Physical Medicine and Rehabilitation Service of the Veterans Administration Outpatient Clinic in Boston. We were impressed by the number of elderly people who were referred to the clinic for treatment. We also noted that some staff members were unwilling to accept the idea that the chronic elderly were being helped by prolonged treatment and rehabilitation; the feeling was that these patients could not receive sufficient benefit from treatment. At first, some pressures were applied by some physicians and therapists to discharge patients even though the latter felt that further attention was warranted. The commonest progress note stated, "maximum possible benefit" or "no further improvement expected."

Because of disparate reactions between patients and therapists in some of these cases, we launched an informal appraisal of the situation. We carefully observed what went on in the clinic and discussed attitudes or reactions toward therapy and therapists with some of the patients. In addition, we reviewed many of the patients' records. We became thoroughly convinced that for a number of them, continued treatment was definitely needed for a longer period than had been previously anticipated.

In essence, we regarded the concept of maintenance therapy as a fifth phase of medicine. The other four are prevention, diagnosis, treatment, and rehabilitation. This book is an elaboration of our concept of maintenance therapy. We highlight its need as well as some of the methods to carry it out, and we subscribe to the idea that even on a maintenance basis, medicine holds great promise for the aging.

JACOB L. RUDD
REUBEN J. MARGOLIN

CONTENTS

MAINTENANCE THERAPY
FOR THE GERIATRIC PATIENT

Chapter I

INTRODUCTION TO THE CONCEPT OF MAINTENANCE THERAPY

JACOB L. RUDD AND REUBEN J. MARGOLIN

IN THE writings and speeches given by the editors to various medical and allied groups, an effort was made to examine the concept of maintenance therapy as it applies to the present-day treatment of the aging patient. With increasing recognition that the future will require more attention to the needs of those with multiple chronic disabilities, maintenance therapy becomes strategic in treatment. Maintenance problems of the patient are beginning to demand more and more of the professional's time. For this reason, more knowledge, interest, understanding, and research are necessary to make the practice of medicine and its allied areas more comprehensive and current as it applies to chronicity and aging.

It was felt that two articles written by the editors, "Maintenance Therapy in Physical Medicine: Relation to Rehabilitation of the Chronically Ill" and "Maintenance Therapy in Nursing Homes," present an appropriate introduction and expression of their perception of maintenance therapy. These two articles are therefore being presented in this chapter.

Maintenance Therapy in Physical Medicine: Relation to Rehabilitation of the Chronically Ill*

Since World War II, the Physical Medicine and Rehabilitation Service has generally been recognized as a powerful force in rehabilitation. Traditionally, such therapeutic practice has been

---

*Adapted from the article which originally appeared in the *Journal of the American Geriatrics Society*, vol. XII, no. 6 (June), 1964.

based on the idea that some sort of benefit—social, vocational, physical or mental—would accrue as a result of treatment. The impetus for this program stemmed from the once pressing need to deal with the large number of handicapped World War II veterans who required restoration to their maximal capacities. Fairly recent (current) trends indicate the emergence of a new program designated *maintenance therapy*. It should be applied along with, and sometimes take priority over, routine short-term rehabilitation procedures.

Maintenance Therapy

Definition

⌈By *maintenance therapy* is meant therapeutic measures which will retard deterioration in patients who are chronically ill by either slowing or arresting the process, albeit temporarily. This concept is important, since more and more patients belong to the group requiring such therapy.⌋ Because many of the other services in the Veterans Administration Outpatient Clinic are also concerned with the problem of maintenance management, a multidisciplinary approach can be used to make the program effective.

Significance

In the Physical Medicine and Rehabilitation Service, as in many of the other services, maintenance therapy is of special significance for the following reasons:

1. The disorders of older persons for which treatment is sought are more likely to be chronic.
2. Many elderly patients return to the Service periodically for treatment because of a greater tendency to recurrence of the old pathology.
3. The Physical Medicine and Rehabilitation Service has traditionally been geared toward definite improvement and early recovery, but now there is need for a more embracing outlook in order to include the maintenance concept.
4. The majority of veterans attending the Outpatient Clinic

suffer from osteoarthritis, chronic back disorders, arteriosclerosis, hemiplegia, multiple sclerosis, or some other
neurologic, orthopedic, or cardiovascular disease. In each
of these situations a prolonged schedule of frequent
treatments is necessary—usually with minimal positive
results even when continued for fairly long periods.

5. Treatment for the long-term patient in Physical Medicine
   and Rehabilitation is considered an essential adjunct to
   the total treatment process furnished by other specialties
   concerned with geriatric or chronically ill patients.

From past experience it would indicate that maintenance
therapy should be classified as intermediate between *habilitation*
and *rehabilitation*. *Habilitation* is concerned with eliciting the
maximal response from the handicapped patient with reference
to the demands of daily living. Because of the severity of the
handicap, it is generally a limited response. *Rehabilitaton* is
primarily devoted to restoring the patient to physical, mental,
social, and economic usefulness commensurate with his abilities
or disabilities. Maintenance therapy involves encouraging the
patient, within his limitations, to enjoy to the fullest whatever
life has to offer at his current physical or mental level.

Background

In the field of medicine, the concept of maintenance therapy
is both old and new. In the field of psychiatry, the idea has
long been recognized. Electric shock therapy, insulin, drugs,
and psychoanalytic therapy are examples of the methods in use
for maintenance purposes in psychiatric hospitals as well as in
outpatient clinics. A psychiatrist may prescribe electric shock
therapy on an outpatient basis to prevent regression. Tranquilizing medication also has a strong maintenance quality. In other
areas of medicine, such as in the treatment of arthritis or
cardiac disease, maintenance therapy is an established procedure.
Digitalis and salicylates are essentially maintenance drugs for
heart disease and arthritis, respectively. The common use of
physical agents for maintenance therapy has often been frowned
upon because the prolonged program of treatments seems
ineffective.

Development of Programs

Attitude of Personnel

One of the problems in developing a prolonged therapy program is the attitude of the personnel. It is fairly difficult for people working with such patients to become enthusiastic when little or no visible progress can be observed over a long period of time. In fact, it is not uncommon for a therapist to become hostile to the program and even feel that some of the patients may be malingering. Although this attitude is understandable, it is not desirable because the patient's progress can be jeopardized. Stanton and Schwartz (1) have demonstrated that when therapists have negative attitudes, treatment of the patients may be affected adversely; patients do not have to see open expressions of hostile attitudes to know that those attitudes exist. Schutz (2) has emphasized the importance of therapist and patient having reciprocal need-satisfaction patterns for therapy to be effective. Barron (3) also has pointed out how sensitive patients are—sensitive not only to the therapist's feelings about them but also to the manner in which he uses the modalities. Barron stresses the compatibility of role interactions as an essential factor. In other words, a therapist, whose emotional need for therapeutic accomplishment is frustrated by the lack of definite evidence of progress as traditionally measured, communicates this dissatisfaction nonverbally as well as verbally to the patient who reacts by also responding in a negative fashion. Inservice training has been utilized in the hope that personnel will be aided in their understanding of the intrinsic values of a maintenance therapy program as well as its relationship to rehabilitation.

Periodic Evaluation

It is contended that if the chonically ill patient feels the need and gives good reasons for continuance of therapy it should not be discontinued even though tangible effects are not obvious. The tendency is to discharge such a patient with a notation of "no improvement" or "uncooperative." If the patient contends that he is being helped by treatment, it is valid to consider his views as an index of improvement. However, in order to dispel any impression that these subjective reactions are the sole criteria for continuation of treatment, it should be emphasized that a semiannual evaluation by the referring physician is required. The subjective reactions of the patient and the objective evaluation by the referring physician, the psychiatrist, and the chief physical therapist should constitute the basis for the decison as to whether treatment should be continued or discontinued.

Attitude of Patients

The philosophy of maintenance therapy raises many interesting questions which admittedly can only be answered by future extensive research: Why, for example, do some patients come to the clinic regularly, whereas others with a similar disorder do not return or come in only once or twice? Is there not an implication here that the treatment or the clinic, for some persons, has not only a physical but also a psychological value? It is important to explore what would happen if treatment were discontinued on these patients over their objections. These speculations need not be purely theoretical. Many patients have asserted that discontinuance would mean an increase in disability and hospitalization. The following comments are typical:

1. "This treatment helps keep me going. I couldn't walk around to do my work without it."
2. "Treatment controls my pain and stiffness."
3. "I wouldn't be able to sleep without treatment."
4. "When I don't get my treatment I become irritable and have to take more pills."
5. "I would be a dead pigeon without treatment."
6. "Take my treatment away and you'll have to save a hospital bed for me."

These statements reflect some of the discouraging reactions to be expected of the patients if they are refused continued treatment. When admission to the hospital is the alternative, it becomes costly to the community and often traumatic to the patient. A significant number of patients receiving long-term therapy are employed, so hospitalization means a loss of employment as well as a loss in terms of self-esteem. It has been experienced that when such patients are discharged they sometimes engage in fantastic maneuvers, including the use of friends, outside physicians, and political influence, in an effort to get treatment reinstated.

Psychological and Physical Values of Maintenance Therapy

It should be clearly recognized that there are both psychological and physical values in prolonged treatment. This duality is not unique. Each of the values is equally important. The rapidly developing field of psychosocial medicine has established the importance of social and psychological influences in general medical and surgical cases (4). There is no question that maintenance therapy provides some psychological support. Patients have indicated this in their own words. The following are examples:

1. "It has helped me to adjust to my condition."
2. "It has given me perspective."
3. "It has given me hope and helped to maintain my morale."
4. "It has helped me to live better in the community, at work, and at home."
5. "It has helped to overcome a feeling of loneliness through socialization with others in the clinic."
6. "It has helped give me a feeling of worth since I have had a chance to help other patients."
7. "It has filled me with a deep sense of gratitude because of the kindness and understanding of the staff, which I felt was of considerable help to me in making the disability bearable."

These benefits suggest that therapists must be constantly alerted to the importance of their role in providing psychological support. Without this awareness the therapeutic effects of physical medicine may be diminished or even neglected. The evidence further suggests that opportunities for socialization and for mutual help through this process is an important avenue of psychological treatment. Not infrequently the therapist and the physician are unaware of these intangible factors. What may seem insignificant to us may be of major importance to the patient. Levin (5), in his study of depression in the aged, contended that many community relationships which are considered minor may actually be of great importance. The same holds true in a therapeutic relationship: what appears to be a cursory factor can be of major sustaining value for a particular patient.

Criticisms of Maintenance Therapy

A common argument against prolonged treatment is that it fosters dependency. Dependency may or may not be fostered, but is it necessarily an evil? Dependency is a very complex dynamic phenomenon with both positive and negative values. For example, if a patient is dependent upon a treatment which helps to maintain him on his job or helps him to participate in civic affairs, then this kind of dependency cannot be considered as a deleterious force but as a facilitative one. Admittedly, the ultimate goal of medical treatment is to make the patient independent (6), and effort should be expended toward this ideal. It should be recognized, however, that certain persons are endowed with fragile egos which contribute to their being dependent personalities. To attempt to move these people to complete independence would be to destroy them. The task in these cases is to utilize the dependency features in a positive and constructive manner so that the patient can make a reasonably satisfactory physical, social, and occupational adjustment.

Relationship to Rehabilitation

It is well to reemphasize that maintenance therapy is not expected to be curative. An attempt is made to keep the aged and/or chronically ill patient functioning to the limits of his capabilities. Not infrequently, treatment helps diminish pain, stiffness, discomfort, and disability. Atrophy, edema, and adhesions may be minimized. However, progressive deterioration is always a danger. Very often the patient recognizes the inevitability of the degenerative process but at the time is grateful for the fact that after treatment there appears to be a loosening of the joints, an increased range of motion, and an ability to perform more of the activities of daily living, despite obvious infirmities. One patient characterized this phenomenon by the unusually perceptive statement, "Treatment helps me, but I'm getting worse."

The removal of all handicaps is not expected, but occasionally an unexpected improvement and recovery occurs. In cases in which there is evidence of rehabilitation potential, every effort is directed toward the realization of rehabilitation goals. At this point, cooperation with other services is crucial because the patient may require concurrent medical, psychological, social, and vocational evaluations.

Case Reports and Comments

The following two case abstracts illustrate some of the under-lying situational dynamics characteristic of maintenance therapy patients. What is most significant are the perceptions of the patients.

Case 1

J. H. S. was a seventy-four-year-old male. His case was diagnosed as follows: Psychoneurosis and anxiety; osteoarthritis of lumbar spine, sacroiliac joints and left shoulder; bronchitis.

He has received continuous treatment for some or all of these disorders in the Outpatient Clinic since 1919. On several occasions he had been admitted to the hospital, but his treatment had been primarily on an outpatient basis. He was married and his wife was still living. He had worked for twenty-five years on a farm and then had had several jobs in municipal departments.

COMMENT

This patient considered treatment crucial to his well-being. Within the previous few years he had stopped work because the joint pains were too severe. He asserted that he would not have been able to work as long as he had without these treatments. In the past when he couldn't come to the clinic, he could get heat treatment at home. He felt that even when he didn't work, the treatment kept him active; without it he would "stiffen up." He looked forward to treatment because, when not working, it got him out of the house and he could talk to people. It helped to pass away the time. He stated that "you don't have to lay down and die" because you are somewhat incapacitated. Chatting with other patients helped him put things in perspective. He thought it was good to talk to other patients because "we help each other out." When some other patient would complain about aches and pains, he would tell him, "You are getting old." Somehow this seemed to make the aches and pains more acceptable. Many of the patients tended to joke about their complaints and even about impending death. In a way, this helped them to accept the inevitability of their handicaps. This patient seemed to understand that there was no miraculous cure for his illness, but he appreciated whatever relief could be secured through treatment. He was grateful that the staff gave of its time, energy, and understanding. He was convinced that without treatment he might not even be able to get around.

Case 2

C. L., a fifty-three-year-old male, has osteoarthritis (chronic) of the dorsal spine and both sacroiliac joints and a conversion reaction. He was a veteran and since World War II had been treated for arthritis by a regular schedule of pills and "shots." Treatment in physical medicine consisted of luminous heat to the lower back, with postural and extension exercises. Because of obesity he was periodically given a weight-reducing diet—with little success. This patient had no delusions, no hallucinations, no psychomotor retardation, and no flight of ideas. He had been married twice, the first marriage ending in divorce. He claimed to be happy with his second marriage which had lasted for seventeen years; there were two children by this marriage. At one time he had been a professional boxer and currently was training boxers. Occasionally he worked as a locker attendant in a bathhouse.

Comment

Mr. C. L. believed that heat treatments furnished relief from aches, pains, and stiffness of the joints and that exercises kept him from getting stiff. He enjoyed talking to other patients and tried to help them by encouraging them to keep going. He often felt depressed and frustrated about the futility of his life. He stated that if he didn't get this treatment he would "get crippled up" and would have to enter the hospital; this would cost him his life and he would "just waste away." With treatment, he could, to some extent, work within his field of training boxers. "Some of us patients wouldn't know what to do if we didn't have a place like this clinic. His part-time work as a locker attendant was not strenuous. Nevertheless, he felt that without treatment he would be unable to handle even this sedentary job. When pain in his neck or back became unbearable, he used home treatments with heat, liniments, and castor oil. His philosophy was to keep moving, keep exercising, and stay out of the hospital "unless you need it." By staying out of the hospital, a little bit of human dignity was retained; it "permits me to do some work." Treatment helped him mentally in that he was convinced it brought some relief. Helping other patients seemed to benefit him. By coming to the clinic he developed a philosophy of life which made him realize how wonderful it was to be able to help another patient. As he expressed it, "A lot of patients used to come in and I would say, 'follow me' and they would have some hope and follow me." He felt that the staff was quite understanding, and he was grateful for their help.

Summary and Conclusions

A report is presented on the physical and psychological impact of maintenance therapy in physical medicine as well as the relation to rehabilitation of the chronically ill. The attitudes of the patients (illustrative case abstracts are included) and of the staff are discussed in emphasizing the benefits of maintenance therapy in long-term treatment programs.

The concept of maintenance therapy is not new, but it has many novel features. It is an essential part of treatment, and its value should not be ignored. The main point stressed in this article is that maintenance therapy has not only physical but also important psychological values. This fact was brought home repeatedly to the editors by patients who indicated that if certain social and psychological needs were not met, their existence would be meaningless. In fact, many intimated that rehospitalization would be necessary to achieve these ends if maintenance therapy were not possible in community settings.

Commentary

This article gave a definition of maintenance therapy which is by no means conclusive or ideal. As more attention is devoted to this area, there is bound to evolve a more precise interpretation of the concept through a process of modification and refinement. Also stressed was its relationship to rehabilitation and the fine, sometimes almost indistinct, boundary between them. A later section of this book elaborates upon the role of physical medicine and rehabilitation.

*Maintenance Therapy in Nursing Homes**

Introduction

The increasing number of geriatric patients requiring nursing care has hightlighted the need for a nursing bed service in many medical areas, including the Veterans Administration. A Department of Medicine and Surgery circular states that in order to implement Section 2 of Public Law 88-450, which is titled "Nursing Home Care in Non-VA Facilities," funds will be made available for thousands of selected veterans who may be placed in Veterans Administration or non-veterans nursing care beds (7). Included in the bill is a provision for increased cooperative relationships between the Veterans Administration and proprietary nursing homes.

This paper is a continuing report of a study on some of the aged patients referred to the Physical Medicine and Rehabilitation Service by physicians in the Veterans Administration Outpatient Clinic. Many of the older veterans sent for treatment are often given maintenance therapy in the outpatient clinic. Others, seen by physical therapists in the home, as home-bound cases, have been receiving a form of coordinated homecare program of maintenance therapy which attempts to conserve,

---

*Adapted from the article which originally appeared in *Nursing Home Administrator,* (November-December) 1965.

preserve, or even develop the individual to his maximum. A number of the home-bound as well as some other handicapped and aging veterans now on outpatient care may eventually be considered as potential candidates for an expanding nursing home care, at present carefully regulated in Massachusetts by several public agencies (8). The Physical Medicine and Rehabilitation Service has been interested in assessing whether or not our present medical procedures are helping in delaying deterioration and so maintaining some stabilizing influence in the chronic diseases suffered by that group of potential candidates. The Service is also interested in assessing whether or not the present maintenance procedures should be expanded to include more occupational, educational, exercise, manual arts, recreational, as well as some light work therapy.

This article touches on the use of active physical medicine maintenance measures as it affects present outpatient, handicapped, aging veterans in general, with some additional thoughts on whether or not some of these methods may be sufficiently useful in the handling of those who are admitted to nursing homes. It attempts a renewal of interest and a reappraisal of the old problem, with an attempt to eventually find a more satisfactory treatment as an outgrowth or improvement on the older, more conservative methods.

Although the Veterans Administration proposed to have some of the Service-connected veterans placed in certain veterans or private nursing homes, it is to be done only after the patient has been admitted to, evaluated at, and secured the approval of the staff of a Veterans Administration Hospital.

Can we help the newly placed veteran in the nursing home by supplying long-term physical medicine procedures which might result in better skilled attention and in fewer complaints of neglect or lack of interest? More information regarding the physical capability of some of these older individuals will be gathered. Will they secure benefit or will they be harmed by a mild, moderate, or even a fairly progressive, somewhat strenuous, exercise activity? Whether such exertion for many of the aged nursing home patients is advisable must be evaluated. It is felt that exercise therapy may be, in some ways, as important an ingredient in maintenance therapy as it is in a more complete sense, the most significant aspect of physical education.

How some of the emotional shock experienced by veterans going into nursing homes for the first time may be eliminated will be determined. Can a more favorable climate by the use of recreational programs and activities of daily living as well as some work therapy be created?

In the Veterans Administration, the Physical Medicine and Rehabilitation Service has since 1948 helped care for the long-term chronically ill "intermediate" patient who needed an indefinite period of hospitalization with rehabilitation. On the other hand, the veteran domiciliary patient, usually better able to take care of himself than the custodial patient and not expected to be confined to bed, also required "a preventive type of care to retard physical and mental deterioration"(9) as well as to diminish the likelihood of being transferred back to a hospital. The above observations were included in a statement as long ago as 1948 by Dr. A. B. C. Knudson, National Director of the Veterans Administration Physical Medicine and Rehabilitation Service program.

In view of the well-known increasing need for the prolonged treatment of almost all the older handicapped individuals, maintenance therapy is assuming a more prominent role in the total therapeutic regimen for chronically ill patients, whether they reside in their own homes, a chronic hospital, a domiciliary, or in a nursing home.* Almost all private physicians, nursing homes, or hospitals, as well as outpatient clinics handling geriatric cases, have to find some sort of solution for about the same problem, namely, one necessitating more prolonged attention, more detailed consideration, better understanding, and real dedicated effort.

---

*Sometimes in geriatrics, as in other specialties, we see some of these patients and say to ourselves or associates, "What's the use?" Apropos of this is a story told of Sir W. Osler, the famous physician, who once put this problem to a young intern. An expectant mother is tubercular. Her first child was born blind, two others died at birth, another was deaf and dumb. The last was tubercular. The father has the pox. "What do you recommend?" "Terminate the pregnancy," said the student. "In that case," said Osler, "You would have terminated Beethoven." (*Globe Man's Daily* story)

The frequently heard statement that mental health and re-habilitation is "everybody's business" holds true especially for "everybody" conducting or working in a nursing home on the multiple physical, mental, and social problems of the geriatric patient.

Definition

Maintenance therapy has been defined by the editors as a treatment method which utilizes therapeutic measures which may help impede the deterioration in patients (who are in more or less static state, though chronically ill) by either slowing or arresting the aging process, albeit temporarily. In a comprehensive medical or surgical program, long-term dynamic maintenance therapy, which may help in slowing down the rate of retrogression or help in temporarily stabilizing the pathological processes, may be considered a fifth stage following four other, better known, stages in medicine, namely, 1) prevention, 2) diagnosis, 3) treatment, and 4) rehabilitation (10). Traditionally, rehabilitation differs from maintenance therapy in that the former is expected to produce a more or less definite lasting improvement in a comparatively short time. In maintenance, the therapy given may be not too unlike that noted in a comprehensive skilled rehabilitation program, but it extends over a long period of time. The results may be static, disintegration may be only a little delayed, and the most that can usually be expected is some slight degree of improvement. Unless persistence plus optimism are present in large doses, the results can be discouraging.

Much of what is meant by maintenance may be considered synonymous with other comprehensive skilled care in a nursing home. Any type of maintenance may be viewed as *the* primary consideration in nursing home care, as the first and the most significant stage, skipping entirely the previously noted first four stages so important in the earlier phases of general medicine and surgery: prevention, diagnosis, treatment, and rehabilitation.

Aging

In a recent seminar, a World Health Organization group of experts on the prevention of premature aging (among them participants from twenty European countries) said that a person between forty-five and fifty-nine is "middle aged," between sixty and seventy-four is "elderly," between seventy-five and eighty-nine is "aged," and over ninety is "very old." Changes which occur physiologically in the elderly, aged, and very old include among other things, calcium deficiency, loss of protein and nitrogen, a lowered basal metabolic rate with lessening of oxygen consumption, hardening arterial walls with impairment of elasticity, and diminution in some or all of the diameter of the blood vessels. It has been said that there is a decrease in all organ functions starting at about the age of thirty years which continues its decline from that age on. In about the eighth decade the breathing capacity may diminish as much as 60 per cent, while nerve conduction may decrease as much as 20 per cent (11). These, as well as other organic changes, are believed to be due to an inability of the aging organism to replace aging or dying cells. According to Mahler (12), however, neither intelligence nor creativity decreases with age.

Recuperation from physical and psychological stresses becomes more difficult as aging progresses. The resiliency in recovery from most of the conditions which befall old age, such as the upper respiratory diseases (pneumonia, asthma, emphysema, bronchitis, tuberculosis), the cardiovascular, metabolic, orthopedic, neurologic, or from any of the other abnormalities found in the elderly, is definitely slowed.

Physical Activity

In spite of increasing age, increasing physical activity for many of the more or less handicapped patients is a procedure which may help improve circulation, lower cholesterol, and produce a feeling of well-being, in general, if kept within tolerance (13). The lack of an appreciable amount of exercise may lead to an increase in osteoporosis as well as in the more commonly encountered stiffness and soreness of joints and muscles. If isotonic exercises are inadvisable, more attention may be devoted to the isometric tensing activities popular with many physical educators and safer, in many ways, than the employment of heavier resistances in the regular range of muscular movements.

The idea that more activity than was formerly thought possible for some of the older individuals is desirable if it follows "the pattern of a progressive series of rhythmical nonstop endurance exercises" has been stressed in articles and books by Dr. Thomas K. Cureton (14), former Professor of Physical Education and Research at the University of Illinois, now in charge of their Physical Fitness Research Center; Dr. Edward L. Bortz, past president of the American Medical Association, who stated that exercise is "the master conditioner for the healthy and major therapy for the ill"; and Dr. Herman K. Hellerstein of the Cleveland Clinic, Western Reserve University, who has been exercising some of the older postcoronary patients (mentioned in an article by Mitchell) (15). At the Veterans Administration Center, Togus, Maine, a warm therapeutic pool gymnastic program for the mentally ill geriatric patient is found to relieve stress and to provide an opportunity to increase the action of all muscles and joints, to learn swimming skills, and to practice the activities of daily living (washing, dressing, and such), as well as to participate in individual and group activities such as the playng of games in the water (16).

With increased exercising there is expected to be in a proper diet a greater need for the amino acids, with a lesser need for fats and sugars. Usually considered helpful are hormones, occasionally vitamins A and D, more often thiamine, ascorbic acid, and riboflavin as well as such minerals as copper, cobalt, zinc, and iron.

Conditions for Which Patients Are Admitted

The individual who is referred to a nursing home is sent because of any one of a number of chronic illnesses, often a cardiovascular-renal disease (includes various stages in the narrowing of the coronaries, cerebral vessels, peripheral vessels, kidney and other circulatory conditions and leads in the causes of death); cancer; respiratory conditions (bronchiectasis, emphysema, asthme, lung tumors); diabetes (with its numerous complications); rheumatoid or osteoarthritis; malnutrition; fractures, especially of the neck or the femur as well as other orthopedic problems including the fairly common thinning of the bone or osteoporosis; injuries, tumors or spondylosis causing damage to the spinal cord, sometimes resulting in temporary or permanent paraplegia or quadriparesis; multiple sclerosis; Parkinson's disease; and psychoneurosis or psychosis; all of which may be included among the more frequently encountered pathology found in the chronically ill or aging.

When treatment is needed for the nursing home patient, it is often of the type which requires, in addition to a well-balanced diet to combat malnutrition, such drugs as digitalis, the vasodilators, sedatives, or narcotics for cardiac maintenance; antibiotics for infections; insulin for diabetes; estrogens or androgens for hormone deficiency and/or osteoporosis; thyroid tablets for hypothyroidism; and cortizone preparations, if needed, for a few of the skin or collagen diseases or for temporary relief of an arthritic condition. Simple progressive relaxation, though not used often enough in the attempt to relieve tensions, seems to be helpful at times and may even be an effective substitute for sleeping pills.

There is some need in nursing homes for tranquilizing medication under medical prescription. According to Dr. Wolff (17, 18), who pioneered in geriatric psychiatry, some older psychotic patients who are disturbed, excited, uncooperative, and hostile (often precipitated by a recent physical illness) have responded with fairly good results to tranquilizers. He further stated that antidepressive drugs have also been successful in certain cases such as those suffering from chronic brain syndrome associated with cerebral arteriosclerosis or senility in which there is reactive depression. Finally, he pointed out that energizing drugs have proved of value in apathetic, listless, and regressed patients suffering from partial disorientation. Many nursing home administrators have voiced the opinion that these new drugs have helped in the treatment and management of the patient.

Increasing Need for Maintenance Measures

With the admittedly exploding geriatric population there is more need for long-term care, whether it be by the previously mentioned private physicians, the chronic disease hospitals, or the home care programs. Long-term custodial, nursing, or restoration maintenance treatment dedicated to helping as many aged individuals return to their community, home, or foster home better prepared for living is the ideal approach to the problem. A few may even start some part-time sheltered work or learn hobbies in a rehabilitation workshop.

The paramount goal, initially, is to preserve the existing level of the physical state and, with help from other specialties, the mental and social status of those individuals. The objective is not a simple one. There have been instances when physicians have complained that, though they were able to bring some of their patients to an optimal level of functioning in hospitals, they sometimes saw them deteriorate soon after they were discharged from an active hospital rehabilitation program and placed in nursing homes, because of a failure to get an early start on the required maintenance attentions needed. Whether or not this assertion is true is not within the authors' province to determine. However, recognition must be given to the fact that, because nursing homes are dealing with an aging population plagued with multiple disabilities, a measure of deterioration is inevitable.

Resistance to Change

People in general tend to resist change. With geriatric patients, resistance to change is an even more important factor in their struggle for survival than with the younger individual. To make matters worse, patients carry with them into the nursing home the stereotype and misconceptions of many of the lay public, the principal one being that a nursing home is a place where you go to die. Orientation of the patient for admission to the nursing home is absolutely essential before any sort of a therapy program can begin. Without such preparation, patients have been known to display a variety of emotional reactions ranging from feelings of rejection, acting-out behavior, or even a marked depression associated with inertia.

A more serious consideration is the possibility that mortality rates may increase within the first three months of admission unless appropriate maintenance measures are taken. There is some research evidence on this point (19, 20). These studies suggest that the combination of the patient's perception of the nursing home as a symbol of death, as well as the magnified disruptive effects on the change of environment, tend to enhance the mortality potential. The studies further emphasize that mortality upon entrance does not necessarily depend on chronological age or physical status (21). Furthermore, psychotic or near-psychotic patients seem to be the ones with the highest death rates after relocation to a nursing home (22).

Physician-Hospital-Nursing Home Cooperation

It is important to recognize that for the most effective maintenance therapy, continuous patient evaluation is required even though the condition is considered chronic, for although the condition is chronic, it does not necessarily mean that it is static. There are subtle changes which have a continuing impact upon the patient's physical and mental status. Then there is, of course, the ever-present danger of periodic, acute flare-ups which frequently require emergency medical care.

A basic step in a nursing home maintenance therapy program is the establishment of a good relationship with the private physician. A close hospital-nursing home cooperative relationship is also needed. Diplomatic and expedient approaches to achieve this goal are necessary. Instead of mutual accusations of unwillingness to work with one another, as is often the case, all parties should get together to determine the channels for back and forth transfer or observation so that the patient's medical needs can be taken care of as they arise. Charles I. Cragg, former Dean of the Harvard Graduate School of Business Administration, wrote that trying to determine "Whose fault was it?" is a complicated issue, one which is essentially unanswerable and one which cannot be asked safely. It is a profoundly disturbing issue which at the very least produces waste, and more commonly produces tragedy (23).

The physician, the hospital, or the restoration center authorities should evaluate a nursing home thoroughly before placing a patient in it. Before referring a patient, the hospital staff should know the ability of the nursing home personnel to carry out skillfully their therapeutic objectives. This approach would obviate any need for a physician to criticize a nursing home's failure to maintain a patient's physical, emotional, and social condition. On the other end of the cooperative spectrum, nursing home officials should become acquainted with the patient in his home or hospital setting before admitting him to their nursing home. If the orientation and preparation process for transfer were initiated with the doctor or in the hospital, admission trauma with its deleterious consequences would be negligible or nonexistent.

Quite essential to the maintenance program, as to other programs, is the free flow of communication. Many hospitals are especially lax in this respect. Communication lacks do not make sense if it is expected that the nursing home do a superior job in the care and maintenance of the patient.

If the premise is accepted that nursing home care functions best in close working relationship with the hospital and/or private physician, then the nursing home has an obligation to provide the necessary maintenance therapy services to meet patient needs. In some instances it may be necessary to bring into the nursing homes resources which are not already there, such as physical, occupational, exercise, or manual arts therapists to assure maintenance levels compatible with the best medical goals possible for the particular case. Some of this help may be paid for by other public or private agencies.

Case Report

With the anticipated increase of placements from the Veterans Administration into nursing homes, assurance of good care takes on added significance as the following simple but typical case excerpt illustrates:

Case 1

J. D., an aging male multiple sclerotic, was being treated by our Outpatient Clinic physical therapist. The veteran was suffering from loss of function in both lower limbs and one upper. At times the patient became partially disoriented, complicating home treatment. In his home he not only fell frequently but he was unable to fulfill adequately the daily demands of living. A housekeeper was available for only two hours a day, and since the other family members were working, the patient was alone most of the day. Because of the difficulties the patient was experiencing in self-care, the visiting Veterans Administration physical therapist, with the approval of the patient's own private physician, advised referral to a good nursing home. At first the family was reluctant to go along with this recommendation, but after a consultation with the physician and the social worker they agreed to admit him to a local nursing home. The physical therapist from the Veterans Administration Outpatient Clinic continued the veteran on ambulatory activities: passive stretching as well as active and some resistive exercises in the nursing home. As of this writing, the patient's physical and emotional well-being have shown appreciable improvement.

Mental Health and Maintenance

It has been alluded that the application of mental health principles is important to maintenance therapy. In fact, mental health and maintenance are so inextricably intertwined that one could not be effective without the other. In a previous publication, Margolin and Hurwitz (24) pointed out that more than 50 per cent of the clients in nursing homes experience emotional difficulties as their prime concern even though their original diagnoses were physical. The creation of a favorable emotional climate is therefore conducive to encouraging the resident patients to participate willingly in routine as well as in maintenance activities.

In a model nursing home where the emotional climate is good, the eruption of a psychiatric disturbance does not create panic. Instead, there is a willingness to take advantage of the services of a psychiatrist or of other mental health professionals who know how to proceed most effectively with such cases. This sort of approach helps minimize the need for a transfer to a psychiatric institution.

Mental health consultation is urgent in a skilled nursing care home in view of the increasing numbers of geriatric patients being transferred from mental hospitals to nursing homes. The maintenance therapy staff works along with the psychiatrist, hoping to prevent the type of regressive effect of institutionalization which can be brought on by the shock of a change of environment. Because of the significance of the new role of the nursing home in the care and treatment of the geriatric mental client, one of the authors is involved in a study at Northeastern University, under a grant from the National Institute of Mental Health, to evaluate those forces which facilitate or retard the adjustment on placement in a nursing home from a mental hospital and to determine the rehabilitation potential of nursing homes for psychiatric patients. Part of the study will include the assessment of the impact of a therapeutic intervention team (psychiatrist, social worker, nurse, rehabilitation therapist) in minimizing adjustment failures of psychiatric patients in nursing homes.

Additional factors contributing to a favorable emotional climate include wholesome staff relationship patterns with others on the staff, with patients, and with their patient's families. Nutritional management, which is alerted not only to dietary needs but also to the psychological and symbolic significance of food, is needed. Awareness of the therapeutic aspects of cleanliness and odor-free atmosphere, a willingness to accept the challenge of developing recreation, and possibly some form of prolonged rehabilitation as a built-in insurance for the patient's psychological and physical maintenance are other requirements.

In the past the authors have stressed the strategic importance of rehabilitation for geriatric patients (25, 26). Their current position does not eliminate consideration of rehabilitation, in the traditonal sense, in nursing homes. However, since the average age of the nursing home resident is now in the eighties although the patient should be considered as an individual, not as an age or a disease), professionals must still be prepared to turn to that phase in care and treatment which concentrates more on possible gains from long-term goals. For these individuals, with some exceptions, concern can be only with getting them to perform successfully as many of the simple activities which relate to sitting up; getting in and out of a bed or a wheelchair; eating and dressing independently; and when possible, ambulating, with or without braces, canes, crutches, or walkers. In addition, the staff should see to it that range of motion is maintained, that proper bed and wheelchair positioning is not overlooked, and that, in general, good posture is stressed.

Summary and Conclusions

The complex problems of maintenance therapy in a nursing home, primarily concerned with an attempt to prevent deterioration by the use of long-term care, have been discussed with a view to the declared increasing need for nursing home care by the Veterans Administration. Although the distinction between rehabilitation and maintenance therapy seems real to the authors, spelling out the difference has not been an easy task. The following suggested steps are helpful in the successful operation of maintenance therapy in a nursing home:

1. Cooperative relationships between the nursing homes, hospitals, and private physicians.
2. Adequate patient orientation to prevent admission trauma when received by the nursing home.
3. A therapeutic regimen which constructively utilizes drug therapy and nutitional management.
4. Creation of a favorable emotional climate and the application of mental health principles with the aid of a psychiatrist and other professionals.
5. Recreational and long-term rehabilitation programs which are concerned with the patient's physical and psychological maintenance.

Commentary

Stressed in this article were the many complex ramifications of practicing maintenance therapy in nursing homes. As in the original article, the basic significance of physical and psychological measures in maintenance therapy have been described. The value of long-term physical medicine and rehabilitation activities in nursing homes has been pointed out. From contact with nursing homes, some excellent rehabilitation programs have been observed. In one nursing home, the impression was that the rehabilitation program was comparable to those in hospitals. There were prescribed physical, occupational, and recreational therapy; an excellent volunteer program; and most interesting, a patient government which was functioning superbly. Although rehabilitation is being increasingly acknowledged by nursing home administrators as needed, there is, however, still no widespread acceptance or implementation of rehabilitation in nursing homes.

Because of the projected increasing use of nursing homes by the Veterans Administration and under the Medicare bill, the character of the nursing homes will have to change. They will have to meet improved criteria and standards of patient care. There is some indication that many nursing homes at present cannot meet the standards expected by governmental agencies under current medical and legislative developments. On the other hand, in fairness to the nursing home administrators, the improved care required by these new programs could be more readily carried out if sufficient Federal, state, and local funds were allocated to nursing homes for this purpose. There is some indication that at present this may not be the case.

With these introductory comments on maintenance therapy, the various ramifications of the maintenance therapy complex now will be examined in greater detail. Because physical medicine and rehabilitation are felt to be more closely allied to long-term treatment than any other phase of medicine, the exploration will begin with "The Role of Physical Medicine and Rehabilitation in Maintenance Therapy." Maintenance therapy is an active component of every phase of medicine. It is the intent of this book to communicate this message.

REFERENCES

1. STANTON, A. H., and SCHWARTZ, M. S.: *The Mental Hospital*. New York, Basic Books, 1954.
2. SCHUTZ, W.: *Three-Dimensional Theory of Interpersonal Behavior*. New York, Holt, 1958.
3. BARRON, F.: *Creativity in Psychological Health*. Princeton, Van Nostrand, 1963.
4. HALLIDAY, J. L.: *Psychosocial Medicine*. New York, Norton, 1948.

5. LEVIN, S.: Depression in the aged: a study of the salient external factors. *Geriatrics, 18*:302-307, 1963.

6. RUDD, J. L., and MARGOLIN, R. J.: Basic concepts in the rehabilitation of hospitalized aged patients. *J. Amer. Geriat. Soc., 8*:531-536, 1960.

7. *Nursing Home Care in Non-VA Facilities.* Public Law 88-450, Section 2, August 19, 1964.

8. FRECHETTE, A. L., and LEVEY, S.: Massachusetts nursing homes today. *New Eng. J. Med., 272*:1010-1012, 1965.

9. KNUDSON, A. B. C.: Rehabilitation of the chronically ill in the Veterans Administration. *JAMA, 162*:1035-1038, 1956.

10. GEORGE, J.: The general practitioner of the future. *New Eng. J. Med., 270*:1286-1291, 1964.

11. SHOCK, N. W.: Physiological aspects of aging in man. *Ann. Rev. Physiol., 23*:97-122, 1961.

12. MAHLER, S. R.: Aging in man. *Postgrad. Med., 30*:527-536, 1961.

13. SWARTZ, F. C.: What is aging? *J. Amer. Geriat. Soc., 7*:905-910, 1959.

14. CURETON, T. K., JR: A physical fitness case study of Joie Ray (improving physical fitness from 60 to 70 years of age). *J. Ass. Phys. Ment. Rehab., 18*:64-72, 1964.

15. MITCHELL, C.: New cure for sick hearts. *True: The Man's Magazine, 19*:66-70, 1962.

16. MILBANK, F. L.: A therapeutic pool program for mentally ill geriatric patients. *J. Ass. Phys. Ment. Rehab., 19*:52-54, 1965.

17. WOLFF, K.: The disturbed geriatric patient. *J. Amer. Geriat. Soc., 12*:1134-1138, 1964.

18. WOLFF, K.: Geriatric psychiatry. *Geriatric Focus, 3*: No. 22, 1965.

19. LIEBERMAN, M. A.: Relationships of mortality rates to entrance to a home for the aged. *Geriatrics, 16*:515, 1961.

20. FARRAR, M., RYDER M. B., and BLENKNER, M.: Social responsibility in nursing home care. *Social Casework, 45*:527-533, 1964.

21. LIEBERMAN: *op. cit.*

22. FARRAR *et al.*: *op. cit.*

23. CRAGG, C. I.: Whose fault was it? *Harvard Business, 42*:107-110, 1964.

24. MARGOLIN, R. J., and HURWITZ, F. L.: The nursing home administrator and mental health practices in the nursing home. *Nur. Homes, 11*:13-15, 24, 1962.

25. RUDD, J. L., and MARGOLIN, R. J.: Basic concepts in the rehabilitation of the hospitalized aging. *J. Amer. Geriat. Soc., 8*:531-535, 1960.

26. MARGOLIN, R. J., and HURWITZ, F. L.: Rehabilitation: the number-one need in the nursing home. *Nurs. Homes, 12*:7-8, 26, 1963.

Chapter II

THE ROLE OF PHYSICAL MEDICINE AND REHABILITATION IN MAINTENANCE THERAPY

JACOB L. RUDD AND REUBEN J. MARGOLIN

E VOLVED in the last few years is the firm conviction (almost an axiom) that in the treatment of the aging there is an ever-increasing relationship between long-term maintenance therapy and physical medicine and rehabilitation (1, 2). For those geriatric patients with multiple disabilities requiring long-term treatment, the relationship is a crucial one. An attempt is made to enhance the well-being of the patient by the use of the usual therapeutic modalities which are part of physical medicine and rehabilitation for the usual length of time, but then, if sufficient relief is not obtained or is temporary, long-term attention must be instituted.

As an over-all general perspective, maintenance therapy is considered to be a fifth phase of medicine. It follows, in a fairly logical sequence, four other phases: prevention, diagnosis, treatment, and rehabilitation. This attitude does not overlook the fact that maintenance may be required as part of or after other types of medical and/or surgical treatment as well as rehabilitation.

Costello and Tanaka (3) felt that the definition of rehabilitation for the aged should include the concept of maintenance. They asserted that "Rehabilitation for the aged needs redefinition. Since few can be restored to gainful employment, for most the goal must be maintenance activity to prevent deterioration. . . . Rehabilitation is aimed toward increasing mental and physical activities and maintaining current faculties so they can live as

28

close to normal as possible with their disabilities. Maintenance rehabilitation is designed to prevent deterioration that accompanies sedentary life. . . . Emphasis should be placed on long-term and maintenance rehabilitation carried on without regard to the element of time to effect correction of factors precipitating admission and restoring persons to society."

Note that mention is made of the need for both physical and psychological measures for maintenance. This point is worth reiterating. Some rehabilitation medicine personnel tend to think only in terms of the physical activity without paying enough attention to the psychological benefits or consequences.

The 1952 Proceedings of the International Congress of Physical Medicine (4) issued a strong statement recognizing the importance of psychological forces: "Most elderly people are suffering from multiple pathological processes, some of them discrete. One of the most important problems is loneliness. Group approach is necessary to deal with all the factors involved. Pathological, sociological and psychological factors must be treated first; then they can be rehabilitated."

REHABILITATION THERAPY

What are the essential elements in physical medicine and rehabilitation which contribute to maintenance therapy? They consist of a variety of activities covering a wide range from the simple to the more complex and sophisticated. In general, a well-rounded rehabilitation program would include some or all of the following therapies: 1) physical therapy, 2) corrective therapy, 3) occupational therapy, 4) recreational therapy, 5) industrial therapy, 6) manual arts therapy, 7) vocational counseling and 8) casework through social service. Veterans Administration hospitals, which are more fortunate than most state or private institutions, usually have trained specialists in each of these therapies.

In some institutions there are individuals who are multipurpose therapists, combining in one person a wide diversity of activities characteristic of the specialty therapies. This individual is generally trained for proficiency in one therapy but usually has sufficient knowledge of other therapies to develop an acceptable rehabilitation program. The outstanding characteristics of the multipurpose therapist should include a dedicated sense of commitment and an ability to get things done unhampered by jurisdictional disputes. The latter may occur when there are a few trained specialists who may cherish the prerogatives of their therapy over the welfare of the patient. In the rehabilitation of the geriatric patient, a multipurpose therapist who is acquainted with many of the therapies can, with the help of aides, perform a useful function when, as in most nursing homes, elaborate rehabilitation programs with diverse therapy specialists are neither available nor financially possible.

Brooke (5) pointed out that the care of our fellow man is part of our American heritage. He viewed the contribution of physical medicine and rehabilitation as helping to relieve pain, develop functional capacities when possible, encourage the family to reestablish a home for the patient if feasible, retain the patient in as dignified a situation as possible, and thus make what remains of the span of his life more bearable, regardless of the progression of disability. Rehabilitation of the body is not the only, or in some cases the most important, aspect of medical care. The dignity of the mind and spirit should always be upheld regardless of the ravages of disease. To achieve this goal, rehabilitation was geared toward the following:

1. Relief or control of clinical symptoms.
2. Strengthening and training of residual capacities.
3. Establishment of attitudes—motivation.
4. Self-care training.
5. Family-patient postdischarge planning.
6. Development of a vocational interest.
7. Disposition of some cases from the hospital to the home or to chronic care institutions in order that prolonged hospitalization in an acute facility be avoided.

The above program exemplifies the many ways in which physical medicine and rehabilitation can contribute to maintenance therapy. One could go a step further than developing a vocational interest by using work therapy as part of a vocational rehabilitation service and thus doing everything to return the handicapped individual to employment. A number of patients over sixty years of age, many of whom had not worked for years, were found to respond magnificently to various phases of vocational rehabilitation. They were returned to employment even though plagued continually by their multiple disabilities.

Where rehabilitation programs are large or are increasing in size, the multipurpose therapist will find difficulty in functioning effectively. In most Federal or state institutions where there are specialists from many different rehabilitation therapies, the involvement of more personnel in rehabilitating the patient requires the team approach. Krauss (7) suggested that the team approach is vital to providing services to meet all aspects of the problems of disablement. Teamwork must begin as soon as possible because of the tendency in the older patient to give up as soon as he realizes he has a chronic impairment. The team approach for the elderly is, however, more easily verbalized than practiced. Sectional debates must not interfere with the progress of treatment. It is a major responsibility of the rehabilitation coordinator to see that maximum benefit is received from the therapies offered through an integrated approach.

Physical Therapy

Physical therapy can help meet the problem of long-term treatment for the chronically ill by the temperate use of physical agents. Physical agents include the employment of the usual modalities such as infrared; hydrotherapy; hydrocollator packs; the various diathermies; ultrasound; massage; galvanic and sinusoidal currents; passive, active, and resistive exercises; and the activities for daily living. Treatment for the chronic individual is not too unlike that given for many cases with acute conditions. The main difference lies in the diminished dosage tolerated by some of the chronically ill and aging, due mainly to impairment of circulation, sensation, or of both. The duration of a particular treatment session is usually less than that required for the younger individual, while the number of applications may have to be extended over months or even years.

A principal objective in physical therapy is to secure the optimum circulation in the involved portion of the body. Other associated objectives include the diminution of pain, stiffness, soreness, and swelling. Exercises are geared toward increasing muscle tone and strength as well as maintaining or augmenting flexibility. Release of contractures may be helped by gentle stretching as well as by exercising the antagonists of the contracted muscles. By devoting attention to maintaining the tone and strength of weakened abdominals, gluteii, and erector spinae muscles either by isometric or isotonic exercises, postural deformities may be combatted.

Because occlusive vascular difficulties increase with aging, the Buerger-Allen active exercises may be introduced into the treatment regimen. These exercises are used in an attempt to increase the peripheral circulation by postural means. They involve simple movements which elevate the extremities, such as doing foot and toe exercises in bed and resting in bed with lower extremities in a horizontal position for about five minutes. These exercises are done to tolerance for about thirty minutes, twice daily.

Care and maintenance of the feet of the aging are often of considerable importance. The elderly are often plagued by the frequently encountered pes planus, with or without the ligamentous strain in the feet and in the legs. Bunions, callouses, coldness of the feet, ulcerations, and gangrene are not infrequently present or occur. In these situations physical therapeutic measures, including some manipulations and the help of any needed medical consultations, seek to furnish relief for the soreness, improve circulation, strengthen the arches, and tighten the ligaments of the feet.

Waugh (8) stressed the idea that physical therapy has, as a basic objective, the physiological maintenance of the geriatric patient. However, his concept of physiological maintenance incorporated a sound body-sound mind frame of reference. Maintenance is achieved by a system of graded, controlled, and supervised activities which prevents adverse physiological changes. This in turn decreases dependency, immobility, nursing, and medical problems. Goals of maintenance in physical therapy were seen by Waugh as follows (9):

1. Maintain tone and mass of cardiac and skeletal muscle and prevent debility.
2. Minimize thrombosis in the gastroc-soleus area.
3. Assist in maintenance and stabilization of vasomotor tone.
4. Enhance nutrition and general body metabolism.
5. Prevent problems secondary to immobilization.
6. Give a sense of belonging and purpose of living.

If the goals of maintenance therapy are to be attained, then physical therapists must not neglect, as some of them still tend to do, the social and psychological factors in treatment. The responsibilities of the physical therapist in this respect have been expressed in cogent terms by Le Guin (10). Not only the physical but the psychological capacities must be assessed. If the patient is overly dependent he must be ego-supported so that he may respond appropriately to treatment. Psychological reinforcement is necessary to restore the patient's self-confidence. Physical therapists are cautioned against establishing unrealistic goals because failure to reach expected goals could be devastating to the patient. It would be better to be content with less-impressive objectives, even if only sufficient to sustain the patient physically and psychologically. Finally, educating society to the psychological and physiological expectations of aging is essential because misconceptions by the public may disrupt the results obtained through maintenance therapy.

Corrective Therapy

Corrective or exercise therapy, no longer a newcomer to the rehabilitation scene, can be of great value in coping with some of the difficult maintenance problems of the geriatric patient. This particular specialty received its greatest impetus during World War II, when the need was great for extra workers to do something for thousands of wounded veterans during their convalescence. Prior to the advent of this specialty, many of the activities conducted by corrective therapists were, and still are, an important part of physical therapy. However, corrective therapy is involved completely in therapeutic implications of exercise in treatment. For a long time, wherever corrective therapy and physical therapy existed side by side in a physical medicine and rehabilitation department, there was, not infrequently, confusion, and even hostility (11). Fortunately, these problems have been quite satisfactorily resolved, and corrective therapy, wherever there is such a department, is accepted as an integral part of the treatment team.

Corrective therapy is the application of medically prescribed activity directed toward the following (12, 15):

1. Maintaining or improving the general state of health of the mentally or physically disabled individual by preventing muscular deterioration, conserving and increasing strength, and strengthening functions of physical residuals.

2. Teaching of activities of daily living, including self-care, health, personal hygiene, training in the use of prosthetic devices, and instruction in functional ambulation techniques and gait training following injury interfering with ambulation.

3. Promoting mental rehabilitation by providing opportunity for socially acceptable creative accomplishments, relief of guilt feelings, expressions of aggressions, and resocialization through physical activity and adaptive sports.

In general, corrective therapy is concerned with the adjustment of the patient to his disability and the development and training of the patient's remaining abilities so that he may lead an adequate enjoyable life in spite of his disability. The most common corrective therapy methods include bed exercises, relaxation exercises, wheelchair exercises, breathing exercises, conditioning exercises, resistive exercises, ambulation exercises, postural exercises, and adapted sports.

Specifically, How does corrective therapy help the geriatric patient to maintain himself? Exercises, properly given, are believed by many physicians to increase the general circulation by increasing the rate of the heartbeat and the force of expulsion of blood throughout the circulatory system. To some extent it is considered to help preserve or even to increase the elasticity of the arteries. It encourages collateral circulation. It helps to maintain and, in some cases, to increase respiratory capacity through increased oxygen intake and utilization. It may maintain the flexibility of muscles while combatting stiffness in joints. All the above are involved in improving physical conditioning as well as tending to contribute to a feeling of well-being.

The authors (16) have previously cautioned that in regard to the aging, the convalescent, or the ill, long-term rehabilitation should be based more on the concept of a "moderate push" rather than on the older "total push" principle. Such moderation encourages involvement in physical, mental, and social activities according to the patient's tolerance level. The disabled and/or elderly are less likely to resist activity when the exercise treatment is one of cautious moderation. In the case of the chronically ill or the aged, only moderate activity is encouraged, not only with ambulation, group calisthenics, and walking, but also with resistances such as the use of weights, the shoulder wheel, the Sargent pulley apparatus, the stationary bicycle, and the punching bag as well as other exercises and the demands of daily living.

Of course along with the physical medicine treatment, the physician sees that the invalid is supplied with whatever is necessary in the way of nutritive supplements containing vitamin C, niacin, and iron. Heart conditions may require tonics such as nitroglycerin or digitalis. Tranqualizers and sedatives are furnished if needed.

By using a "moderate-push-to-tolerance program" over a prolonged period in all the rehabilitation therapies, it is felt that an appreciable contribution can be made to the over-all maintenance aspects in the treatment of the geriatric patient (17).

Occupational Therapy

The previous descriptions of two of the therapeutic activities in rehabilitation medicine are intended to provide some insight into the potential of physical medicine and rehabilitaton for maintenance therapy. Occupational therapy has generally been accepted as a vital ingredient in any rehabilitation program. It is even more important when utilized in the treatment for the aged. In fact, in many situations in which budgetary considerations limit the extent of rehabilitation programs, it is the only type of rehabilitative activity which is functioning. Without occupational therapy activity, physical and mental deterioration in many cases cannot be combatted. An increasing number of convalescent centers and nursing and rest homes are currently introducing occupational therapy because of its high maintenance value

Occupational therapy has been basically defined as an objective type of treatment prescribed by a physician to hasten a patient's recovery from disease or injury or to contribute to his adjustment to hospitalization (18). It includes in its armamentarium a wide variety of activities to meet the patient's physical and psychological needs. Occupational therapy is all-embracing in scope. It employs activities which may be educational and/or recreational. It may deal specifically with arts and crafts, or it may include advanced occupational activities important in prevocational exploration. The two major branches of occupational therapy include preventive or diversional therapy and kinetic or functional therapy.

Occupational therapy goals are in many respects similar to those of physical therapy: They seek to increase the range of motion, restore muscular function, prevent muscular atrophy, and lessen weakness and incoordination as well as improve, in general, the physical and mental state. As with physical therapy, activities for daily living can be taught to the patients very effectively. Geriatric patients often find that occupational therapy provides a more specific meaning to their existence in an institution. The psychological aspects of such an undemanding form of work is a very important factor in helping to maintain the patient. An increasing number of nursing homes and homes for the aged are introducing occupational therapy. More research is beginning to emerge in an attempt to evaluate the effectiveness of occupational therapy in a few of the nursing homes or homes for the aged. More investigation should be carried on in this area as well as on the effects of maintenance physical and occupational therapy for the home-bound.

For a proper evaluation there must be a set of realistic objectives for which to strive. Wolk *et al.* (19) have established the following goals for the residents in the Memorial Home and hospitals for the aged in Brooklyn, New York:

1. Encourage group activity and socialization.
2. Improve the physical status of the patient.
3. Retard further regression and isolation.

In this home the average age of the patient is 83.9 years. Their program is classified as dynamic occupational therapy requiring constant adaptation to meet the changing needs of the residents. Activities range from arts and crafts to the educational and recreational. The program has been well received by the residents. The authorities feel that it is an excellent diagnostic instrument for a continuous recording of the emotional reactions of the residents as it should also be for the physical.

It is interesting that in nursing homes and homes for the aged the possibilities of sheltered workshop programs are more often being explored than ever before. Here again there is a wide range of approaches to the utilization of sheltered workshops in a geriatric institution. In some nursing homes which were visited, a simple type of sheltered workshop was noticed. In these the patients fabricated certain products such as stuffed animals which were sold to visitors, and the patients used the money to purchase more materials. In one nursing home, an ingenious idea was observed: The patients in this institution negotiated with a candy company to have a variety of candy products shipped to the nursing home on consignment. A small store was established within this nursing home to sell the candy for profit. Patients were assigned a number of occupational roles such as salesmen, store manager, and advertising agents. The proceeds from the sale were donated to charity; the patients contributed one-hundred dollars to the local chapter of The American Cancer Society. In another nursing home the patients took the proceeds from the year-long sales of stuffed animals, scrapbooks, and so on and offered a five-hundred-dollar scholarship to a local girl to train in nursing.

A more ambitious type of sheltered workshop in a home for

the aged was described by Roberts (20). A registered occupational therapist was hired, and as part of the occupational therapy program a sheltered workshop was established. Subcontracts were secured from local industries, and the residents of the home worked mornings in the workshop. In the afternoon an occupational therapy program was carried on with an avocational and recreational emphasis. The residents of the home worked diligently and responded enthusiastically to this balanced program. In fact, the demand for participation in this program was so great that they expanded their facilities an additional 3,300 square feet. The sponsors of this program claim that it has proved its value. A large number of patients were involved, and the number of visits to the doctor declined. The aging participants were so busy working that they did not have as much time to be concerned about their aches and pains. One of the major visible effects was the complete disappearance of a depressed atmosphere (21). This experience described by Roberts substantiates in many ways the findings of Peffer (22) and Rudd (23) with the member-employee program as well as their attitude and that of others toward work and workshops (24, 25, 26, 27, 28, 29). Unless meaningful experiences are taken seriously into consideration and provided to individuals who have disengaged themselves from lifelong roles because of retirement or disability, then maintenance problems—both physical and mental—may become quite acute and severe. All are familiar with the histories of individuals who have deteriorated and died shortly after retirement from a life of productivity to one of anonymity and purposelessness.

Educational Therapy

One should not hesitate to utilize any constructive measure or process, be it medical, educational, avocational, or vocational, which would help maintain the patient. The therapeutic value of education for geriatric patients tends to be underestimated. Experts on the functioning of the aging mind now tell us we can continue to learn until the day we die. There are many examples of "students" in their eighties and nineties who learned difficult subjects for the first time. Group discussion on current events, for example, can serve to maintain the geriatric patient's interest in his surroundings.

Hulicka (30) gave a succinct description of the value of educational therapy for geriatric patients. She stressed the importance of providing opportunities to the elderly for maintaining their dignity and worth and of displaying their accumulated wisdom among their peers and with the staff. Geriatric patients have responded enthusiastically to participation in book clubs and discussion groups in which a variety of subjects can be discussed. The program described by Hulicka is fairly characteristic of educational therapy programs for geriatric patients wherever they exist in institutional settings. They are directed primarily toward reducing social isolation, exploring mutual interests, improving emotional climate, and enhancing self-esteem. Even though the cost of this therapy may be high, intellectual stimulation for geriatric patients cannot be neglected, since the loss resulting from such deprivation may be even higher.

Of course there are patients who cannot benefit from educational therapy either because they are too ill or because they are in a too advanced state of physical or mental deterioration. However, the value of this oft neglected therapy for those patients able to profit from it is crucial.

Manual Arts Therapy

As with educational therapy, manual arts and industrial therapy can play a significant role in maintaining geriatric patients. There may be some raised eyebrows when activities involving woodworking, metal working, and printing programs or the placing of patients seventy years of age or older in work situations around the institution are advocated. The objections may include the possibility that working with tools, especially power tools, may be too hazardous or that an industrial therapy work situation may overextend the geriatric patient. There is some validity to these objections, but the risks can be minimized by proper safeguards so that there will be little or no danger present to prevent the physician from prescribing these activities. In previously mentioned articles on the member-employee program and on workshops, the authors have stressed the idea that all activities in physical medicine and rehabilitation, when carried on in moderation for geriatric patients, can contribute significantly to their maintenance.

It is gratifying to note that a number of nursing homes and homes for the aged have introduced manual arts and industrial therapy into their rehabilitation programs. These activities have great therapeutic value for geriatric patients. They require some basic skills and to some extent replicate the productive world outside the institution.

Visits to modern rehabilitation centers for the aged are dramatic revelations. Patients eighty years of age and older are busily, constructively, and happily engaged in a variety of manual arts or industrial-type activities.

Best (31) has called attention to the increasing number of older patients with chronic disabilities who are being assigned to manual arts therapy programs in the Veterans Administration. He noted that even if employment is not feasible for older patients, they would derive great satisfaction from pursuing activities closely related to what is going on in industries outside the hospital.

In the industrial therapy program under the supervision and direction of the authors (32), the maintenance value of work was clearly demonstrated. Many of the patients were in the geriatrics age group but still found work stimulating and even essential to their well-being. They were able to perform successfully in a variety of occupational tasks such as kitchen work, janitorial service, farming, landscaping, furniture repair, painting, and clerical work. Allowances had to be made for those patients who could not work as fast as formerly and who could not work a full day. However, these factors did not detract from the importance which such work had in preventing physical and mental deterioration.

Activities of Daily Living

Probably the most crucial activities in physical medicine and rehabilitation for optimum maintenance of geriatric patients are the activities for daily living. These activities are not the sole prerogative of any one therapy in physical medicine but can be taught by all of them. Activities for daily living are especially central to therapeutic goals in corrective, physical, and occupational therapy. Each of these therapies has created basic functional approaches and imaginative self-help devices to encourage many of the severely handicapped patients to participate successfully in important daily activities.

The aim of this program is basically to restore the patient to independent living by teaching him to cope adequately with the daily demands of life. Specifically, patients are taught to do for themselves a variety of tasks such as eating; dressing; washing; toileting; getting in and out of bed, a wheelchair, or a car, boarding and departing from public transportation; crossing the street; and many other practical responsibilities. It is very difficult for those with normal functioning of their extremities, relatively free from disease and injury, to realize how difficult it is to perform the simple functional tasks which were once automatic. To become independent again requires a relearning of even the simplest movements. It is especially difficult because in addition to the presence of arthritis, general arteriosclerosis or a mild-to-severe neurological disability is not unusual.

In many cases, only a partial restoration of independent living can be expected, but this limited progress in view of the severity of the disability can be considered a significant gain. Even the slightest improvement in motion function and activity results in better patient morale and usefulness.

Rusk (33), a pioneer in rehabilitation, stressed the point that activities for daily living must be practiced in a real-life situation. The training of the patient must be carried out within the limits of his physical and/or mental disabilities and must be inherent to his daily life in the home, at play, or at work if he is able to be employed. He recommended that the training program to teach any specific activity be broken down into three phases: 1) breakdown of the activity into its simplest motions, 2) examples of exercises to be practiced so the motions can be accomplished, and 3) examples of preparatory exercises when the patient is not ready for the exercise itself.

Careful evaluation of a patient's progress in meeting the

demands of daily life should be built into the treatment process from the very beginning. Improvement not only in functional capacities but also in general learning ability and motivation should be measured (34). It is advisable to set up evaluation as a twofold process. One aspect, professional evaluation, would be for the benefit of the physician, the therapist, and others working with the patient. Essentially, this can be considered as a progress report providing a frame of reference for reaching treatment goals. Concerning professional evaluation, a number of measures may be used, including qualitative assessments such as progress notes, and quantitative assessments such as numerical ratings of patients.

The other aspect of evaluation is for the patient's benefit. Many hospitals and rehabilitation centers have some sort of self-scoring system or scorecard which enables the patient to obtain some picture of his progress. Schoening *et al.* believed the scorecard to be an excellent motivational device to move patients forward in their rehabilitation.

A substantial number of patients, despite serious handicaps usually multiple in nature, were surprisingly able to recuperate sufficiently to maintain themselves at adequate functioning levels. In a previously published report (35), two cases were presented to illustrate this point. The first case was a poignant illustration of how medical rehabilitation served as a valuable maintenance therapy agent. The use of the hydraulic lift is one of the best maintenance measures available for the relief of pressure on an incipient decubitus ulcer (36).

Case 1

S. R. was a retired storekeeper, seventy-eight years old. After an automobile accident he was hospitalized for multiple fractures of the pelvis and right leg. In about two weeks' time, the main treatment problem concerned some recently developed ulcers of the sacrum and heel. An overhead crane operated by a hydraulic lift was secured, and appropriate use of this apparatus helped prevent further ulceration of the back and heels; the ulcers which were present began to improve slowly. In about three months, with help from specialists in orthopedics, medicine, dermatology, and plastic surgery, and with continued use of the hydraulic lift, the decubitus ulcers cleared up completely without the extensive skin grafting operations which had been contemplated.

After discharge, despite the serious fractures (which had been followed by ulcerations of the back and heels), he had other disabilities such as anemia, edema of the legs, and heart murmur. However, the patient was able to walk, cook his meals, care for himself, and do light work in his home—including taking care of an oil heater which served two apartments. He is now also able to sweep the floor and when necessary shovel some light snow. He does not stay in bed during the day, eats well, attends meetings when an automobile ride is available, is mentally alert, and requires no medication to sleep at night.

Physical medicine procedures included bed exercises for the strengthening of the upper extremities, attention to posture, early elevation from the bed by hydraulic lift, supported ambulation, and ultraviolet irradiation to the ulcerated areas on the back and heels.

He has and still has several pathological conditions but is not really sick. He had and still has many serious disabilities but is not seriously handicapped.

The second case (37) illustrated that to which has been previously alluded, namely, that an individual with proper care and treatment can return to work even after a long absence from employment.

Case 2

This sixty-nine-year-old white veteran of World War I had been hospitalized for twenty years. His symptoms first developed after he had suffered from business reverses. He had paranoid delusions, had become antisocial, seclusive, and resistant to treatment. Pulmonary tuberculosis was discovered during a routine chest x-ray examination about eleven years after he had been hospitalized as a mental patient. There was extensive bilateral infiltration of the upper lobe, more marked on the left. He was treated by crushing of the left phrenic nerve and was given streptomycin and isoniazid. The condition cleared up satisfactorily over a period of several years.

He was suicidal or assaultive but fluctuated between being over suspicious, noisy, and resistive to treatment and being quiet and cooperative. For a long time he thought that his sputum had some special properties and was unwilling to part with any of it. Insight and judgment were somewhat defective. His mental condition showed little change up to the time at which chlorpromazine was started, approximately a year before his discharge. He changed from a hostile, angry person to one who was much more pleasant and approachable.

In the physical medicine and rehabilitation program he was advanced from occupational and manual arts therapy to an individual industrial therapy assignment. His performance was good, and he showed aptitude as a furniture repairman as well as a greenhouse worker. He was therefore recommended for the member-employee rehabilitation program. At first he resisted attending, claiming it was a plot to keep him in the hospital. After ventilating his fears and anxieties, he accepted a job assignment on the member-employee program as a furniture repairman. His work adjustment was excellent.

He was discharged from the program after four months when a job in the community was secured for him as a greenhouse worker. At the same time he was placed in a foster home about two miles from work. Despite his age, he walked to and from work daily. Both the social worker and the member-employee supervisor, who was a counseling psychologist, conducted close supervision for a long period of time. After living in the foster home for almost two years he requested permission from the employer to convert an unused garage, located on the greenhouse grounds, into living quarters so that he could be near his work. Permission was granted, and he alone performed all the alterations, construction, and painting necessary to convert the garage into decent living accommodations. He has been working for a period of four years and is still "going strong." The patient worked steadily for a period of eleven years (until he was eighty years old). The last information received about him was that he was still working one or two days a week and was also enjoying semiretirement through constructive participation in leisure time activities.

That employment should be considered for all aging persons is not being advocated. Obviously, such an ideal is not possible. However, it is felt that with a selected number of individuals, remunerative employment should be viewed as an integral part of the maintenance therapy program. Indeed, in special cases, even though the patient is retired from his lifelong work, employment is the ingredient which will prevent personality deterioration.

Baxt (8), who described a successful vocational rehabilitation program for the older disabled worker (sixty-five and older), was quite emphatic about the older disabled person's employment potential. He declared that the feasibility of vocational rehabilitation for the older person has been clearly demonstrated. It is not a question of feasibility but rather of 1) how many can be served, 2) how the quality of service can be improved, 3) who can best render these services, 4) what the best pattern of community organization for providing these services is, and 5) how these services can be financed. In his agency (Federation of Employment and Guidance Service, New York City) and based on experience with 1,500 individuals, Baxt reported that for each one-hundred persons, fifteen will drop out before completing service, five will be diagnosed as unemployable, sixty as employable for competitive industry, and twenty as employable in sheltered workshops only (39).

Every physician should have some familiarity with the concept of maintenance therapy. He should also be aware of how physical medicine and rehabilitation contributes to maintenance. Because of the increasing number of aging who are in need of individual treatment (long-term and otherwise), and who because of Medicare and other health measures will eventually be able to receive treatment, it is especially vital today to have this knowledge. The only way this goal can be accomplished, as Knudson (40) intimated, is to incorporate the teaching of such concepts into the medical school curriculum. Some medical schools have already pioneered in this respect. It is the authors' hope that more will follow.

REFERENCES

1. RUDD, J. L., and MARGOLIN, R. J.: Maintenance therapy in physical medicine: relation to rehabilitation of the chronically ill. *J. Amer. Geriat. Soc.*, *12*:582-588, 1964.
2. RUDD, J. L., and MARGOLIN, R. J.: How maintenance therapy helps patients. *Nurs. Home Admin.*, *19*:49-51, 1965.
3. COSTELLO, J. P., JR., and TANAKA, G. M.: St. Louis chronic hospital program. *JAMA, 167*:7-13, 1958.
4. COSIN, L.: The part of physiotherapy in geriatric rehabilitation. *Proc. Int. Cong. Phys. Med.*, 1952.
5. BROOKE, C. K., SCANLON, T., and GUARINO, G. A.: The role of physical medicine rehabilitation service in the treatment of long-term chronic patients. *Med. Bull. Veterans Admin.*, *19*:307-311, 1943.
6. *Ibid.*

7. KRAUSS, T.; MORELEWICZ, H. V., and DOZORETZ, L.: The role of comprehensive rehabilitation in the care of the geriatric patient. *New York J. Med.*, 55:2331-2335, 1955.

8. WAUGH, J. W.: Objectives of physical medicine and rehabilitation in a chronic disease and geriatric facility. *J. Amer. Geriat. Soc.*, 10:522-525, 1962.

9. *Ibid.*

10. LE GUIN, K. W.: Some aspects of gerontology: their importance to the physical therapist. *J. Amer. Phys. Ther. Ass.*, 44:348-352, 1964.

11. HAWKINS, W. B.: Corrective therapy in the physical medicine rehabilitation services. *J. Ass. Phys. Ment. Rehab.*, 5:13-14, 1952.

12. *Manual of the Association for Physical and Mental Rehabilitation, Incorporated.* 1964-1965.

13. YOUNG, C. H.: *Directional Goals for Clinical Therapy Experiences for the Association for Physical and Mental Rehabilitation, Incorporated.* New York, 1958.

14. MONTAVANO, L. F.: Preliminary survey and analysis of the educational and professional background of the corrective therapist. *J. Ass. Phys. Ment. Rehab.*, 7, 1953.

15. BERNER, L., and TAUBER, A.: Physical education in medical practice. *J. Amer. Ass. Health Phys. Educ. Recreation*, 24:32-35, 1953.

16. RUDD, J. L., and MARGOLIN, R. J.: Basic concepts in the rehabilitation of the hospitalized aging patients. *J. Amer. Geriat. Soc.*, 8:531-535, 1960.

17. DAVIS, J. E.: Evaluation and planning for the elderly psychiatric patient. *Geriatrics*, 18:238-246, 1963.

18. *Manual of Occupational Therapy.* Chicago, AMA, 1943.

19. WOLK, R. L.; SEIDEN, R. B., and WOLVERTON, B.: Unique influences and goals of an occupational therapy program in a home for the aged. *J. Amer. Geriat. Soc.*, 13:989-997, 1965.

20. ROBERTS, S.: Occupational therapy and sheltered workshops program in a program for the aged. *J. Amer. Geriat. Soc.*, 10:532-534, 1962.

21. *Ibid.*

22. PEFFER, P. A.; MARGOLIN, R. J.; STOTSKY, B., and MASON, A.: *Member-Employee Brochure.* A collection of papers by the staff of the Veterans Administration Hospital, Brockton, 1956.

23. RUDD, J. L. Physical medicine and rehabilitation in the member-employee program. *Arch. Phys. Med.*, 38:505-508, 1957.

24. RUDD, J. L.: The Massachusetts Rehabilitation Commission (Medical), Department of Industrial Accidents. *New Eng. J. Med.*, 248:366-369, 1953.

25. RUDD, J. L., and FEINGOLD, S. N.: A work adjustment center in vocational rehabilitation. *Arch. Phys. Med.*, 40:29-34, 1959.

26. RUDD, J. L., and FEINGOLD, S. N.: Medical and vocational cooperation in a geriatric workshop. *J. Amer. Geriat. Soc.*, 8:349-359,
1959.

27. MARGOLIN, R. J.: A comparative analysis of member-employee programs in Veterans Administration hospitals. *Amer. Arch. Rehab.
Ther.*, 7:114-122, 1959.

28. LEIBERMAN, J. M., and KNUDSON, A. B. C.: Compensated work as
therapy. *Amer. Arch. Rehab. Ther.*, 12:13-23, 1964.

29. WINICK, W., and WALSH, F. X.: Community hospital industrial rehabilitation program. *Ment. Hosp.*, 15:147-150, 1964.

30. HULICKA, I.: Educational therapy for geriatric patients. *Amer. Arch.
Rehab. Ther.*, 11:95-100, 1963.

31. BEST, E. E.: Manual arts therapy in our changing time. *Amer. Arch.
Rehab. Ther.*, 9:20-24, 1961.

32. RUDD, J. L., and MARGOLIN, R. J.: Industrial therapy in a member-
employee hospital. *Amer. Arch. Rehab. Ther.*, 4:225-230, 1956.

33. RUSK, H.: *Rehabilitation Medicine.* St. Louis, Mosby, 1958.

34. SCHOENING, H. A.; ANDEREGG, L.; BERGSTROM, D.; FONDA, M.;
STEINKE, N., and ULRICH, P.: Numerical scoring of self-care status
of patients. *Arch. Phys. Med.*, 46:689-697, 1965.

35. RUDD, J. L., and FEINGOLD, S. N.: Medical and vocational cooperation
for the aging. *J. Amer. Geriat. Soc.*, 5:263-270, 1957.

36. RUDD, J. L.: The hydraulic lift for decubitus ulcers. *J. Bone Joint Surg.
Amer.*, 37-A:202-203, 1955.

37. BAXT, R.: Vocational rehabilitation of the older disabled person: a
successful program. In *Rehabilitation of the Older Disabled Worker
—the Academician's Responsibility.* R. J. Margolin and F. L.
Hurwitz (Eds.), United States Department of Health, Education, and Welfare, Vocational Rehabilitation Administration, Washington, D. C., November, 1963.

38. *Ibid.*

39. *Ibid.*

40. KNUDSON, A. B. C.: Rehabilitation of the chronically ill in the
Veterans Administration. *JAMA*, 162:1035-1036, 1956.

Chapter III

PHYSICAL FITNESS IN MAINTENANCE THERAPY FOR GERIATRIC PATIENTS

JACOB L. RUDD AND REUBEN J. MARGOLIN

INTRODUCTION

PHYSICAL fitness has become an integral part of maintenance therapy. Long-term treatment and physical fitness are inextricably bound together because it is difficult or impossible to maintain one's health without paying serious attention to the benefits of long-term, even though usually moderate, physical activity.

Recently there has been a resurgence of interest in and a more optimistic view of the effects of physical activity on the geriatric patient. Previously, the approach to increased physical exertion with the aged was regarded with some ambivalence bordering on skepticism. The well-known experiments with conscientious objectors during World War II dramatically demonstrated the harmful effects of inactivity even upon the normal, healthly, young adult (1). Subjects showed significant losses in blood volume, calcium, nitrogen, vitamins, and so on. Muscle atrophy due to disuse as well as generalized weakness was noted after only a few weeks of recumbency. As a result of these experiments there was a widespread tendency toward bed exercises and earlier ambulation even after a serious illness of radical surgery.

Mead (2) described this trend as an end to a century of the abuse of rest which has persisted despite the lack of scientific justification for such practice. He described a study in which normal volunteers were immobilized in plaster casts for six weeks. The effects were catastrophic and like the previously mentioned experiment included the following:

1. Vascomotor instability and tremor.
2. Impaired blood pressure and homestatic mechanisms.
3. Negative calcium and nitrogen balance.

Similar results were noted when women, following delivery, were subjected to prolonged confinement. Sudden death from a pulmonary embolus was a not too rare autopsy finding. A thrombophlebitis would sometimes result in permanent swelling or disability of a lower extremity. Now that the period of confinement has been drastically shortened, the occurrence of such fatal or untoward results appears to have diminished. Mead concluded that most Americans at work or at play are inclined to be somewhat averse to strenuous exertion. More physical activity is needed by most of us. This is believed so even with the geriatric patient (3).

AGE AND ACTIVITY

That an individual should become less active because he is growing older is a fallacy. Rudd and Margolin (4) emphasized that some energy should be expended but on a moderately balanced program of activity commensurate with the existing tolerance level. Man is by nature an active creature. Diminished activity can and often does lead to an inertia which inevitably results in physical and mental deterioration. Not only does physical activity, especially the judicious use of exercise, aid in preventing mental and physical decline, but it often increases a person's stamina despite increase in his number of years.

It is universally agreed that precautionary measures should be taken against overexertion. If there is definite shortness of breath, tightness of chest, a feeling of nausea, or marked fatigue after exercises, these signs should be regarded as danger signals that exercise has been carried too far or that the organism is unable to cope with the additional strain. Incipient symptoms such as those just described should be sufficient warning to cease such activities or to bring them within moderate bounds. Failure to heed could result in circulatory disturbances such as peripheral vascular involvement, coronary attacks, cerebral anemia, or respiratory distress.

Riccitelli (5) has pointed to inactivity as an important geriatric problem. Stated another way, exercise, as an ingredient of maintenance therapy, is needed for geriatric cases. Riccitelli urged us to take a more realistic concept of the aging process. He vigorously asserted that therapeutic exercise combined with good nutrition could help solve many vexing geriatric problems. Functional capacity (both mental and bodily vigor) would be maintained, vascular tone would be improved with a speed-up of circulation, cardiac and pulmonary function would be improved, and physiological involution would be delayed. Morehouse and Miller (6) asserted that physical exercise can make a significant contribution in preventing premature aging and in some cases preserve some of the physical characteristics of youth. That exercise defers old age and helps to prolong life was expressed as far back as the early part of the twentieth century (7).

An interesting case was described by Dill and Wasserman (8). A physically fit person at age ninety had carried out throughout his lifetime a regime of exercise which kept him physically fit despite multiple handicaps which required several serious surgical procedures including laparotomies for intestinal obstruction, a cholecystectomy, and a transurethral prostatectomy. Physical fitness tests revealed that this person, physiologically, was nearer sixty than ninety. This finding underlines a concept which is very important for all who work with the aged to understand: There may be a wide discrepancy between physiological, chronological, psychological, and sociological ages. It is understood that a person might be either physiologically younger than his years or older than his chronological age. At the same time he might be psychologically immature but sociologically adequate because of his ability to perform satisfactorily in the occupational world.

The prevailing opinion among authorities today is the acceptance of the idea that regular exercise, in moderation, is essential to good health in old age. Recent research by a Russian investigator (9) on 550 persons between the ages of forty-five and seventy years indicated that exercise led to considerable improvement in their subjective conditions. Cardiovascular findings, including the electrocardiagram, showed that improvement had occurred and that the adaptability to standard effort was enhanced. The electroencephalogram showed that the functional state of the cerebral cortex was increased. Oxygen saturation of the blood increased. Protein fractions of lipid metabolism were normalized in patients with arteriosclerosis. The adrenal cortex and other areas of the endocrine system functioned more normally. Exercises were carried out in gradually increasing dosages, with differentiation in range and intensity. The factor of moderation was stressed as extremely significant. The general conclusions were that exercises are of great value in maintaining health during this age period.

GENERAL BENEFITS OF MAINTENANCE ACTIVITY

Claims concerning the benefits of exercise for the geriatric patient have ranged from the cautiously optimistic to the widely enthusiastic. Some of these claims tend to reach beyond the reality potential of the therapeutic benefits of exercise. Although exercise appears to be important to health, it is unlikely that it will prevent the eruption of active disease processes. Physical fitness, for example, is not considered to be much help as protection against infections.

The authors are attempting to show that moderate progressive "resistance until discomfort detected" activities such as walking, running, swimming, and so forth, do help maintain the essential vital functions of the body, especially the cardiovascular system. Appropriate exercises can also be of some direct benefit in the treatment of most of the neurological, psychiatric, and orthopedic conditions prevalent among the aged. To the extent that this is true, exercise is an essential ingredient of maintenance therapy.

Gerontinos (10) stressed the disabling complications which can occur in healthy individuals who limit their physical activity. Atrophy of muscles, contractures, incoordination, as well as osteoporosis could be the unfortunate result. Chronic disabilities plague a large number of people in our society, yet they are able to function satisfactorily in daily living because they engage in a sensible program of physical activity which involves conditioning of the muscles of the body.

MAINTENANCE EXERCISES

There is a variety of physical fitness approaches which appear to be effective in maintaining the geriatric patient. Some of the more common exercise methods, such as the isometric or isotonic and including the moderate progressive resistance approach, have been considered in the field of preventive geriatrics. In hospitals, patients may actually develop disabilities which are primarily traceable to inactivity, immobility, and prolonged bed rest and which could not be blamed on the conditions for which they were admitted.

A preventive geriatric program should be instituted with bed patients. The nature and extent of the bed exercising program would vary with the kind of disability present. In the arthritics or the postoperative orthopedic cases, bed positioning and range-of-motion exercises would be helpful. Posture, resistance, and stretching exercises to extend and/or abduct the stump help to prepare postsurgical amputees for ambulation with a well-fitted prosthesis.

Krauss (11) in a recent book described another kind of preventive program which is pertinent not only for the young but also for the geriatric patient. In his opinion, the majority of the estimated twenty-eight million Americans who suffer from backache (a large number of whom are over sixty-five) are underexercised and overtensed. His prescription for a bad back or for preventing one is a simple but intelligent exercise routine.

Rudd and Margolin (12) reached similar conclusions on the importance of exercise for back cases a few years ago when they had the opportunity to deal with 340 patients who complained of back difficulties. Many of these patients were suffering from what were diagnosed as "tension backaches" or "postural strain." In these cases, attempts were made to relieve the muscular and nervous tension by establishing correct body mechanics and teaching progressive relaxation. In a surprising number of selected cases, manipulation or stretching was performed and proved very helpful.

Precautions must be taken against treating all back conditions as purely functional. Many with osteoarthritis or with disk protrusions are problems which may require drugs, physical medicine, or even surgery as basic therapeutic agents; yet even in these cases the inclusion of an exercise program can be important in first improving, then maintaining, physical fitness.

Isometric and Isotonic Exercises

Isometric and *isotonic* exercises of various types have been employed in most of the geriatric treatment programs. Each of these has been used in various therapeutic activities for a number of years, and each has its enthusiastic supporters. The basic difference between the two types is that *isometric* exercises rely principally upon muscle tensing. In essence, isometric exercises lead to the development of tension without shortening of the muscle. *Isotonic* exercises, on the other hand, involve active exercises which go through the full range of motion. Morehouse and Miller (13) described isotonic exercises as the application of a force through a distance which results in the performance of work.

Recently, more interest has been evidenced on the use of isometric exercises for the older individuals in the geriatric treatment programs. Some feel that it is easier to encourage most patients to engage in physical activity which does not appear to require a heavy expenditure of energy. Many patients resist active exercise programs because they cannot reconcile the idea of their multiple handicapping conditions with active exercises as a beneficial therapeutic agent. Proponents claim that muscle tensing is a safe, quick method of securing the benefits of exercise for the maintenance of health. Allen (14) indicated that isometrics may be encouraged with patients eighty years or older. By this method not only is muscle tone maintained, but many believe that muscle strength is greatly increased.

Although there is value to isometric exercises properly used, isotonic exercise cannot be neglected in the treatment of the geriatric patient. Isotonic exercises, carefully regulated, progressive to tolerance, is the most effective of the methods for exercising the heart muscle. Whether it be used for the normal young individual or for the aging, sick, or the convalescent, it will aid most in the maintenance and improvement of the cardiovascular pulmonary complex. This philosophy reflects the authors' conviction that regular isotonic activities adapted to the individual's capacity, both in sickness and in health, is important.

The appropriate use of physical activity has made appreciable contributions to the strength of the weight lifter (15) who uses isometric exercises as well as to the postoperative bed patient who requires a safe type of muscle building without motion as part of his management. Exercises have been given credit for speeding up the recovery of surgical and maternity patients, for aiding in the prevention of thrombophlebitis, emboli, kidney stones, calcium loss and other mineral loss from bone (osteoporosis), and for helping to restore physical and mental health to elderly invalids. Such "corrective therapy" plays an important part in the rehabilitation of those who have had poliomyelitis, stroke, arthritis, and fractures, as it does in patients with a variety of other neurological or orthopedic disorders (16).

Moderate Resistances

Finally, a word about heavy resistance versus moderate resistance efforts: The authors have never advocated heavy resistance exercises for the geriatric patient, the ill, or the convalescent. Many investigators believe that almost any method, whether it be heavy or moderate resistance, isotonic or isometric, is as good as any other (17). More realistically, an assessment must be made of the individual's condition to determine which approach or combination of approaches would be most beneficial for him. With rare exception, heavy resistances would be overtaxing or might even be damaging to most of the elderly. Moderate resistance movements, on the other hand, can have a direct relationship to the daily activities of the aging.

Rudd (18) has previously stated that under ordinary living conditions (for minimum daily tasks or requirements of daily living), an expenditure of energy roughly comparable to the physical effort involved in a moderate amount of weight lifting is required. Heavy resistances for the aged or the convalescent, therefore, are not at all necessary or advisable in most exercise sessions. By the use of a moderate resistance-repetition exercise, with its inherent, associated, built-in purposeful simplicity and avoidance of undue strain, an individual who is in poor general condition because of age or is weakened by disease (but still needs to expend some effort daily) can receive the benefit of a safe form of conditioning by brisk walks, jogging, bicycling, or swimming.

Value of Exercise in General

The value of exercise as a preventive, conditioning, or remedial force in the treatment of various medical conditions for the younger patient has been well documented by some of the investigators previously mentioned here as well as by a number of others. A well-planned but moderate resistance exercise program can also help restore the ill geriatric patient to independent living and can help reduce the number of nursing, medical, or ancilliary personnel needed to care for them. Graduated exercises and physical fitness programs have been prominently mentioned as aids in the recovery of those with certain types of cardiovascular conditions (coronary, angina, peripheral vascular diseases, cerebral vascular accidents, and hypertension) as well as with neurological, arthritic, and psychiatric states. It is surprising how many physicians still encourage their convalescing and/or aging patients to lead a sedentary existence when actually the opposite, with reasonable discretion, is indicated.

Exercise and Heart

Dr. J. W. Morris (19) of the British Medical Research Council concluded from his researches that regular exercises should be included as a "way of life" which would promote health in middle age and that heart disease may be in some degree a deficiency disease—a deficiency in regular physical activity throughout life. Since the cardiovascular system is so strategic to the health of all other organic systems in the body, it is most important that exercises for such a condition be prescribed and supervised in order that maximum benefit be secured and harm avoided.

More has been recently written about the importance of physical fitness for cardiovascular conditions than perhaps for any other ailment. The best-known exponent of this point of view has been the eminent cardiologist, Dr. Paul Dudley White. In the preface to Guild's (20) book on physical fitness he wrote: "As a cardiologist I have concluded from my practice of more than forty years and from current scientific investigations that keeping fit also delays in all probability the onset of crippling rusting of the arteries themselves which we call atherosclerosis, the great epidemic of today." Jokl (21) substantially agreed with this position when he stated that exercise exerts a protective influence against degenerative cardiovascular disease.

White has not neglected the importance of physical fitness for patients over sixty-five. In a talk (22) given some years ago, he mentioned a study of two-hundred patients with coronary thrombosis after sixty-five and five-hundred with angina pectoris. He concluded that for those who took better care of themselves by being physically active, the prognosis for recovery was much better than for those who neglected this phase. He felt that the rehabilitation program for the cardiacs was both therapeutic and preventive and that for the older patients it was invaluable in any maintenance procedure.

Straube (23) pointed out that the most important measure in rehabilitating aged cardiovascular patients is to increase physical training slowly in sufficient dosage and to avoid sudden overexertion. He maintained that this sort of careful exercising helps increase coronary reserve and collateral spread and tends to lower cholesterol levels. He advocated additional measures, including respiratory training to be given along with physical training.

In findings reported to the scientific sessions of the American Heart Association (24), the Health Insurance Plan of the Greater New York Study revealed that a male leading a physically active life has a two to three times better chance of surviving a heart attack than someone less active. He also has a much better chance of escaping the attack in the first place.

Fox (25) has summarized some of the recent research on the value of physical activity to cardiovascular health. His review of investigations on the relation of physical activity to cardiovascular health and the important mechanisms involved suggested that physical activity is beneficial. More important, the evidence he presented indicated that recent activity is more valuable than activity earlier in life and that even a light or moderate amount of physical activity may be significant to the health of the individual. Such an attitude points the way for more extensive studies which are sorely needed to provide additional information regarding the mechanisms involved in exercising and how they benefit function.

His detailed review of the literature covered some of the investigations which were carried out on the relationship of physical activity to ischemic collateral vascularization, to adiposity-obesity, to lipids, blood coagulation and fibrinolysis, to hypertension, functional circulatory insufficiency, and especially to myocardial efficiency. Of considerable interest has been the apparently beneficial effect of regular exercise on the aging as indicated by the outstanding example of Joie Ray (26).

Interest in exercising has expanded to include not only those who are "normal" in their aging but even to some of those who have had heart involvement, hypertension, or diabetes. The reluctance to give exercises to the elderly, despite the fact that many appear to thrive on it, is more common than one would suppose. It is especially so if the elderly have, or have suffered from, any pathology of the cardiovascular system. This attitude is being broken down gradually by a number of highly respected medical investigators as well as by those in the field of physical education.

Edward Leroy Bortz (27), Thomas K. Cureton (28), Herman K. Hellerstein (29, 30), and Paul D. White (31) were among the first investigators to indicate that exercise was helpful for the aging individual. Two of these investigators have shown that many of the victims of coronary attacks could, after a satisfactory convalescence, embark on a gradual progressive-to-tolerance regimen of activity which would eventually include running or swimming for increasingly greater distances. After a few months of slow progression to more vigorous exercises, it was observed that some appreciable improvement usually resulted in the follow-up testing (32) of the pulse and blood pressure of the hypertensive or cardiac candidate for cardiovascular conditioning. Increased endurance accompanied by a feeling of improved well-being was not an unusual result.

The Cambridge Young Men's Christian Association Program

At the YMCA in Cambridge, Massachusetts, the Physical Fitness Council has been involved, since the early 1960's, in a dynamic program for physical fitness utilizing a gradual progressive-to-tolerance approach. Although there is no limit on age, a physical examination and written approval by the candidate's own physician is required before the candidate is accepted.

The first conditioning workout which is started in a day or two is divided into three simple areas: 1) the warm-up, 2) the work, and 3) the tapering off. When exercise is done in this sequence, most of the participants proceed from low gear levels of exercising for fitness to medium, and from medium gear levels to high without appreciable discomfort.

All the candidates for the conditioning program had had in their preliminary examination a graphing with the heartometer which, to some extent, measures "work" (33, 34). Comparison is made of the size, shape, and rate of the person's pulse on the heartograph, before and after exercising. Although the heartometer does not measure stroke volume, it is at present the best and most useful instrument available to the Cambridge YMCA to measure cardiovascular fitness.

When cardiovascular fitness is improved by many months of moderate, progressive "resistance until discomfort detected" activity, the above-mentioned shape, size, and the slowing of the pulse rate shown on the heartograph indicated better heart filling as well as more forcible contraction of the ventricles. Of additional importance are the systolic and diastolic blood pressure readings taken when seated, standing, and after jumping in place for one minute. Evidence is sufficient to indicate that after attaining fitness, a definite diminution is not infrequently found in a high systolic and is usually accompanied by a more important decrease in the diastolic blood pressure of many of the hypertensives. This lowering may be maintained by individuals who have more or less gradually become mile runners even after their running activities have stopped.

The chances of keeping the blood pressure lower is best for those who train regularly on the gymnasium track. Blood pressure lowering appears to depend fundamentally on a maintenance program of exercising which should be continued as long as feasible so that the definite benefits noted in many of the cases may be maintained. Even for the severely disabled, conditioning may be helped by a program of exercising to tolerance (35).

Two of a large number of cases indicating the beneficial effects of exercise on patients with hypertension are here recorded:

Case 1

A sixty-year-old male participant on the first visit gave a history of hypertension and showed a blood pressure reading of 165/100. After six months of gradual, progressively increasing activity (mostly running), his pressure was reduced to 140/90. This lower reading has remained around this figure with continued exercising. For him, routine gymnasium activities usually consist of a mile run, two to three times a week. In his present state of conditioning this is considered a moderate degree of maintenance exertion.

Case 2

A forty-year-old male auto salesman started the YMCA program with a blood pressure reading of 190/110. A year later the conditioning had decreased the pressure to 150/80. Although he was not the winner of the event, this same individual was able to compete in and complete a five-mile race held in his home town.

For years the Cleveland YMCA had a fitness program for cardiacs. Based on the program initiated by Thomas K. Cureton, PhD, Director of the Physical Fitness Laboratory at the University of Illinois, the Cleveland program of Cutler and Morris for postcoronaries consisted of graduated walking, jogging, running, swimming, and calisthenics. This program was subsequently evaluated by a cardiologist, Dr. Herman K. Hellerstein of Western Reserve University, who was surprised to find that many of the reconditioned cardiacs were in better condition than the average "normal" users of the YMCA gymnasium.

When the Cambridge YMCA was prepared to start activities

similar to those of the Cleveland YMCA, a letter was sent to a number of physicians who were expected to be interested in an exercise program. On December 14, 1962, the following letter was sent:

> There is considerable interest and curiosity among medical men regarding the effects of the various physical fitness programs. We now have an opportunity to listen to, question, and work with physical educators in order that we may better determine the kind of program best suited for the patients we see.
>
> The questions are: Do these programs improve cardiac efficiency, the aging process, reduce hypertension, and benefit the patient psychologically as well as physically? Which of the programs is best medically?
>
> With these thoughts in mind we have invited one of the top experts on physical fitness, Dr. Thomas K. Cureton, to discuss the latest work done in this area. His discussion 'The Heartometer and its Role in Physical Fitness' will be held on Friday, January 11, 1963, at 4:00 P.M. at the Cambridge YMCA.
>
> You are most cordially invited to attend this session designed specifically for medical men. You are also invited to attend any of the demonstration exercise sessions listed in the enclosed brochure. Very sincerely yours, J. L. Rudd, M.D., Medical Member, Cambridge YMCA 'Physical Fitness Council.'

The Cambridge YMCA program had already been started in the fall of 1961 with the help of the Physical Fitness Council, spearheaded by a dynamic leader, Alexander Melleby, then the Physical Director. On a strictly voluntary basis, a number of interested, dedicated, business and professional men, members and nonmembers of the YMCA made up the council. In less than a year after its formation the Chairman of the Physical Fitness Council wrote:

> You will be interested in knowing that over 200 'Y' members have been tested and, due to the publicity and results that have been obtained, the Cambridge 'Y' has seen its greatest increase in membership in the last twenty-five years. I would like your continued participation in the Physical Fitness Council.

VETERANS ADMINISTRATION RESEARCH PROTOCOL

A study entitled "Will Physical Conditioning Help the Hypertensive and Cardiac?" was projected in cooperation with the Boston Veterans Administration Outpatient Clinic. Statements in the rather ambitious protocol included the following:

The Problem:

To find out whether exercises have definite beneficial effects on heart, lungs, and blood pressure for the normal as well as for the cardiac and hypertensive individual. The validity of the following physical fitness theses will be assessed:

(a) Heart muscle can be strengthened by vigorous rhythmic endurance exercises.

(b) Neither work nor exercise, but the lack of it, contributes to hypertension and coronary disease.

The Method of Study:

1. Questionnaires will be given in which the individual applicant will be asked questions concerning his:

(a) Fitness-Health Activity Type.

(b) Previous Activity.

(c) Personality Type.

2. Tests will be given to help determine:

(a) Efficiency of heart and height of blood pressure as measured by the heartometer.

(b) Weight in terms of bone and fat proportion.

(c) Rating for body measurement and fat measurement.

(d) Vital Capacity.

(e) Balance.

(f) Muscular endurance, power and agility.

This study involves the evaluation of approximately three-hundred participants to further determine the claimed beneficial effects of exercise, especially on the hypertensive, the cardiac, and/or the aging (36).

That the activities program outlined above will increase longevity is not known. Hopefully, the experiment will be continued long enough to help determine whether there is any tendency in that direction. Judging from some of the benefits noted in this particular physical fitness YMCA clinic over the last five years and the resulting lowered blood pressure in some hypertensives (compared to what they had before exercising, without drugs), and according to the longevity ratings of life insurance statistics based on blood pressure, an increased life span appears possible.

EXHIBIT AT AN ANNUAL MEDICAL MEETING

An exhibit on "Cardiovascular Physical Fitness Tests" was presented at the Annual Meeting of the American Congress of Physical Medicine and Rehabilitation in Philadelphia, September 1965. The exhibit was initiated by the VA Outpatient Clinic, Boston, Massachusetts, at the instigation of the Physical Fitness Council of the American Congress of Physical Medicine and Rehabilitation and in cooperation with the Cambridge, Massachusetts, YMCA.

The Cameron Heartometer graph readings on the brachial pulse after sitting, standing, and then running in place for one minute were taken from doctors who served as volunteer patients. A large number of the medical men at the meeting were tested, and the findings regarding systolic and diastolic blood pressures; the pulse rate; and the shorter, higher, sharper, or other changes in the size and shape of the graph of the pulse before and after exercise were explained. Only after they were tested did some of the doctors inform us that they had had at some time one or more coronary attacks. No ill effects were noted from the jumping in place for one minute for any of the former victims of coronary artery occlusion.

The physicians were shown earlier graphs taken at the Cambridge YMCA on those members who had been participating for months in a progressive exercise program of walking, jogging, running, swimming, and calisthenics. The graphs, indicating the changes in size and shape of the pulse and the lowered blood pressure after exercising, were exhibited in greater detail at the Annual Meeting of the American Congress of Physical Medicine and Rehabilitation to physicians who were interested.

Graphic presentation helped to indicate the degree of significant cardiovascular improvement which took place following months of regular exercising. The graphs taken at the first examination of the newly arrived applicant were contrasted with the pulsograph taken months or years later on the same heartometer. Some of the graphs showed, by an improvement in the shape of the pulse wave and especially by the diminution in the height of the systolic and diastolic plateau, that after exercise, high blood pressure was reduced appreciably.

Despite the considerable information secured from the heartogram of the brachial pulse, more accurate information which might be obtained from a better testing machine is being sought. To date, sufficient evidence which would warrant purchasing another type of equipment has not been found. Most of the instruments claimed to be better are, for research purposes, very expensive, very complicated, and, as yet, not sufficiently practical to be a worthwhile substitute for the present machine.

In June 1965, a portion of the VA research progress report stated:

> Since the last report, approximately thirty subjects a month have been checked in preparation for a physical fitness program. The total number now engaged in this study is three hundred. Ten per cent of these cases are in the upper age bracket (sixty to seventy years), another 20 per cent have some hypertension, a few have had a form of heart pathology for which their doctors permit only a mild to moderate form of progressive physical activity.
>
> Results to date support, to some extent, the theory that regular physical activity does have definite beneficial effects on the functioning of the heart, lungs, and blood pressure of the hypertensive and cardiac as well as the average individual, regardless of age. At the Cambridge YMCA where most of our investigations in this field are carried on, eighty-one subjects who were retested after three months have shown a lowered blood pressure, improved circulation, a feeling of well-being, and an increase in work tolerance.
>
> Case reports are being compiled for future publication. We have been in frequent contact with the physical director of the 'Y' to supply the information which contains the findings to date. The case reports will be carefully reviewed and evaluated in more detail as soon as feasible.
>
> The exhibit and testing on physical fitness at the Annual Meeting of the American Congress of Physical Medicine and Rehabilitation, Philadelphia, August 22-27, 1965, was part of a successful multiple exhibit on the general subject of physical fitness.
>
> We are contemplating further investigations on the same group of patients, after they have had anywhere from six months to five years of the physical fitness program, to determine the effect of such a long-term program on the heart, blood pressure, and lungs.
>
> We hope to continue the experiment long enough to be able to form an opinion regarding the insurance claims that the lowering

of blood pressure as well as exercise which puts a strain on the heart and arteries tends to increase longevity.

THE PHYSIATRIST'S ROLE

The testing of the effectiveness of a physical fitness program which may be adapted to the medical rehabilitation effort could be done with little cost to the Government. The facilities, personnel, experience, and techniques used by the Cambridge YMCA Physical Fitness Council may be used to help in the research program. With the help of the facilities and personnel of the Cambridge YMCA, an evaluation of the results of their program on the pulse and blood pressure is planned. This has been seriously attempted in a number of areas. Of interest will be the claimed effect on some of the recently afflicted individuals who are permitted (even encouraged) by their own physicians to go through with such exercise programs (37, 38).

More questions arise than can be answered, but before some of these questions can be answered to everyone's satisfaction, a larger number of hypertensives and cardiacs will have to be carefully checked for longer periods. Of the many queries, convincing replies will be sought to the following:

1. Can the Physical Medicine and Rehabilitation Service in the VA, with the help of physical and corrective therapists, utilize some of the above methods of conditioning?
2. Could the YMCA facilities be used and, in this way, test the VA patients in their gymnasium on a modified community basis?
3. Do the previously medically approved patients, especially the handicapped and the aging, really benefit from physical activity with respect to their cardiovascular status?
4. What is the effect of exercise on longevity?

The editorial by Thomas P. Anderson, MD, in the February 1966 *Archives of Physical Medicine and Rehabilitation* expresses the authors' sentiments:

"There was no revival of interest in the use of exercise in medicine until recent years. With our present emphasis on exercise, we must take care not to repeat the errors of the ancient Greek physicians who placed too much reliance on the gymnasts. If we, as physicians, prescribing exercise, do not give close attention to specific details, it is likely that harmful excesses might result from such exercise or that less than maximal benefit might be expected." Henry Longstreet Taylor, a co-worker with Ancel Keys in the University of Minnesota's Laboratory of Physiological Hygiene, is not too convinced of the benefits of exercise and stated that only four sedentary individuals die of coronaries for every three active men (39).

PATIENTS WITH SEVERE HANDICAPS
Physiological-Neurological

In addition to examining a large number of applicants for the physical program who were average, as well as a few cardiacs and some hypertensives, a number of VA patients who had marked disabilities were tested—paraplegics, multiple sclerotics, and hemiplegics. Some of the handicapped were confined to wheelchairs, some were on crutches, and others used canes for support in ambulation. It was not too surprising to find that many of the seriously paralyzed reacted on the pulsograph as if their cardiovascular status were good. Because the hearts and arteries of the handicapped are usually exercised considerably more than that of the average, active individual, the results were to be expected.

Often a maximum of physical effort is required to insure mobility for a disabled individual. The limited functioning of the involved nerves and muscles necessitates considerably more than average exertion by the remaining skeletal muscles as well as by the cardiovascular mechanism. Any movement involving standing or walking, even between parallel bars, invariably means the expenditure of all available energy in order that the patient may attain the erect position or even a small amount of mobility.

Markedly handicapped hemiplegics, paraplegics, arthritics, and multiple sclerotics, when tested for cardiovascular physical fitness, showed pulsographs indicating that they were in surprisingly good physical condition. On investigation it was amply demonstrated that these patients were the ones who were physically active despite their disability. Most of these individuals must exert an unusual amount of strain on their residual skeletal as well as their cardiac musculature in order to maintain mobility.

The story is told that when President Franklin D. Roosevelt was asked how he was able to keep up the arduous duties of his office without appearing to tire, he replied that he was used to work; it took him months of strenuous activity just to learn to move his big toe. This anecdote illustrates the large amount of effort which had to be expended to obtain even a small amount of mobility. It tends to give a clue in answering the question, Why do so many of the disabled appear to have good cardiovascular response despite their handicap?

For severely disabled individuals, especially those with orthopedic or neurological involvement such as hemiplegia or paraplegia, training in self-care activities and ambulation not only teaches the essential functional activities but provides a foundation of physical stamina to carry out these activities (40). The age of these handicapped patients should not be considered sufficient cause for avoiding instruction in ambulation or in any of the essentials of daily living. In fact, delay may impair health and contribute to poor posture, breathlessness, palpitation after slight exertion, muscular atrophy, or mental fatigue, and may even lead to such serious complications as thromboses, ulcers, or urinary infections.

The concept that early activity after prolonged bed rest (while in bed or sitting up, walking, bicycling, trotting, jogging, and so on) will tend to strengthen cardiovascular adjustment and diminish mental stress has been accepted by many physicians who practice modern medicine. More inactive capillaries are dilated, heart muscle is strengthened, and oxygen is transported more effectively to more tissues.

Diabetes

Too little attention in the past has been directed to the effect of strenuous exercise on the diabetic patient. There is little in the literature which describes the close relationship between exercise and the lessened need for medication or injection which controls blood sugar. Once it was quite generally believed that the influence of exercise in the control of diabetes was not too significant, but this attitude is changing. Alexander Marble of the Joslin Diabetic Clinic expressed the opinion that exercise was definitely helpful in diabetes, since it caused some changes in the blood serum which appeared to have a beneficial metaboliclike effect similar to that of insulin. Some of the research done by Goldstein and Levine (41) tends to indicate the correctness of this statement.

Engerbretson (42) has been doing some interesting research on the effect of exercise in the control of diabetes. He has a special interest in this area, since he is not only trained in the field of physical education but is also a diabetic. Some case reports (including his own which involves exceedingly strenuous mountain climbing) show that exercise, in addition to improving the physical fitness of the diabetic patient, helps to reduce the amount of insulin needed. He established a rigorous training program for himself as well as for other subjects, the effect of which was a definite lessening of requirements in the control of diabetes. His conclusions were derived from the measurement of blood and urine sugar levels and the per cent of negative urine tests.

Mental Retardation

Little concern has been directed to the effect of physical fitness upon mental retardates. The literature reveals a paucity of research on the motor functioning of the mentally retarded (43). Recently there has been a surge of interest in providing physical fitness programs for them. The Kennedy Foundation, as an example, granted funds to the Boston School System to establish a physical education program for the retarded. Many local chapters of the retarded children associations have organized physical education activities because school and community have too often neglected this aspect of their education.

For mental retardates, physical activity has many important implications which have been previously overlooked. Since both longevity and life efficiency are greatly dependent upon the level of physical fitness, it is one of the most essential of the maintenance measures. It is well known that retardates are susceptible to physical and psychological stresses which make them more prone to secondary complications from illness and injury.

Physical fitness activities are also basic to improving motor skills, coordination, and organic power. The more deficient the retardate is in these areas, the greater the benefit he will derive from guided, controlled endurance and/or strength exercises which will help him cope with the demands of daily living. Exercise such as that in games, sports, and rhythmic movements should be carefully used in accordance with the retardate's innate intellectual capacity to perform these activities. Physical activity, correlated with intelligence and combined with emotional considerations, forms the tripod upon which stands the type of long-term maintenance therapy which will provide maximum benefit for the mentally retarded.

Psychiatric Conditions

The value of physical fitness for psychiatric patients has long been recognized (44, 45, 46, 47, 48). Almost all mental hospitals employ physical education as a therapeutic agent. Psychotic patients frequently show lower physical fitness scores on physical fitness tests than so-called normals and psychoneurotics. In fact, one of the greatest dangers in a psychiatric hospital is physical and mental deterioration of the patient. Catatonic patients, for example, suffer the risk of circulatory difficulties which can be very serious. If they remain immobile for any period of time, as many of them do, a condition of stasis characterized by extensive edema of the lower extremities becomes a serious medical problem. This type of passive congestion is usually changed to an active hyperemia by supervised, lower extremity exercises.

As in the case of the mental retardate, physical activity is a basic measure for maintaining well-being but not necessarily for the same reasons. One of the main problems with psychiatric patients is that they have lost contact with or have a tenuous hold on reality. Consequently, resocialization becomes a prime objective in treatment. Physical activity can initially arouse interest in reestablishing or maintaining contact with reality. The patient responds to this process because physical activity excites psychomotor-sensory stimuli which are pleasurable. For the mental patient it may represent a return to the original primitive state in which all responsibility is obliterated and the pleasure principle reigns supreme.

High-level improvement is often maintained because physical activity provides opportunities for release of hostility and aggression through socially acceptable channels. Punching-bag activities afford an illustration of this concept. Explosive and dangerous behavior can be channeled through this medium with a resultant dissipation of violent energy. At the same time, the activity is enjoyable and physically healthy. A heavy expenditure of energy not only provides a cathartic release through nonverbal means, but it also leads to an over-all state of relaxation. An abatement of psychological and physical tensions generally follows the termination of such exhausting activities.

In a recent study the employment of persistent physical activity as a motivating force with aged psychiatric patients has been considered sufficiently significant to be used with success on some of the very regressed, chronic mentally ill (49). Exercises have been used with some of the psychotics afflicted with tuberculosis. The Brockton Veterans Administration Hospital has been one of the pioneers in this aspect of corrective therapy (50). For a number of years, exercises were given to mental patients afflicted with tuberculosis who were being given streptomycin, para-aminosalicylic acid, and/or isoniazid. Originally started on an experimental basis, physical activity became an accepted therapeutic procedure in this hospital as well as in approximately twenty other institutions with tubercular-psychiatric beds. The majority of the psychotics with not too advanced tuberculosis were helped. Physical endurance and appetite appreciably increased.

SUMMARY

This chapter attempted to show that physical fitness is an essential ingredient of maintenance therapy. The attitude of others, physicians and physical educators, toward the value of exercise in helping to develop a feeling of well-being as well as in contributing toward the prevention of cardiovascular and other degenerative disabilities has been mentioned. How physical activity serves as a maintenance measure in patients suffering from various handicaps has been described. The results to date have been encouraging but are not conclusive. Much more research in this area is necessary and is continuing.

REFERENCES

1. KEYS, A.: Effect of bed rest on blood volume of normal young men. *Amer. J. Physiol., 144*:227-232, 1945.
2. MEAD, S.: A century of the abuse of rest. *JAMA, 182*:344-345, 1962.
3. *Ibid.*
4. RUDD, J. L., and MARGOLIN, R. J.: Basic concepts in the rehabilitation of the hospitalized aging patients. *Amer. Geriat. Soc. VIII*, 7:536-538, 1960.
5. RICCITELLI, M. L.: The therapeutic value of exercise in the aged and infirm. *J. Amer. Geriat. Soc., XI*, 4:299-302, 1963.
6. MOREHOUSE, L. E., and MILLER, A. T.: *Physiology of Exercise.* St. Louis, Mosby, 1963.
7. LORAND, A.: *Old Age Deferred.* Philadelphia, Davis, 1912, pp. 248-250.
8. DILL, D. B., and WASSERMAN, K.: Fitness at 90: a new record. *Gerontologist, 3*:135-140, 1964.
9. MOTYLYANSKAYA, R. E.: Some aspects of the scientific investigation of the effect of active exercises in old age. From this symposium. *Vop. Geront. Geriat.,* pp. 221-229, 1962.
10. GERONTINOS, E. M.: The physical fitness requirements of the older disabled individual. *J. Ass. Phys. Ment. Rehab., 18*:105-106, 1964.
11. KRAUSS, H.: *Backache, Stress and Tension: Their Cause, Prevention and Treatment.* New York, Simon and Shuster, 1965.
12. RUDD, J. L., and MARGOLIN, R. J.: Rapid rehabilitation of back cases. *J. Ass. Phys. Ment. Rehab., 6*:9-107, 1949.
13. MOREHOUSE, and MILLER: *op. cit.*
14. ALLEN, J.: The use of isometic exercises in a geriatric treatment program. *Geriatrics, 20*:345-347, 1965.
15. HOFFMAN, R.: *Exercise Without Movement.* York, The Bob Hoffman Foundation, 1961.
16. *Consumer Reports.* October, 1959, pp. 543-544.
17. RUDD, J. L.: A simple resistance exercise method. *Amer. Practitioner, 13*:145-148, 1962.

18. RUDD, J. L.: Moderate resistance exercises. *J. Ass. Phys. Ment. Rehab.*, 5:150-153, 1956.
19. *Consumer Reports. op. cit.*
20. GUILD, W. R.: *How to Keep Fit and Enjoy It.* New York, Harper, 1962.
21. JOKL, E.: *The Scope of Exercise in Rehabilitation.* Springfield, Thomas, 1965.
22. WHITE, P. D.: Heart Disease after Sixty-Five. Address to American Medical Women's Association Board of Directors Meeting, Boston, November, 9, 1956.
23. STRAUBE, K. H.: Rehabilitation in cardiovascular disease. *Z. Aerztl. Fortbild. (Berlin)*, 13:743-747, 1916.
24. Release from the American Heart Association Annual Meeting and Scientific Sessions, 1965.
25. FOX, J., and SKINNER, J. S.: Physical activity and cardiovascular health. *Amer. J. Cardiol.*, 6:731-745, 1964.
26. CURRENS, J. H., and WHITE, P. D.: Half a century of running: physiologic and autopsy findings in the care of Clarence De Mar. *New Eng. J. Med.*, 265:988-993, 1961.
27. BORTZ, E. L.: *Creative Aging.* New York, Macmillan, 1963.
28. CURETON, T. K., JR.: Physical fitness work with normal aging adults. *J. Ass. Phys. Ment. Rehab.*, 11:145-149, 1957.
29. HELLERSTEIN, H. K.: Assessing and preparing the patient for return to a meaningful, productive life. *J. Rehab.*, 32:51, 1966.
30. HELLERSTEIN, H. K.; BURLANDO, A.; HIRSCH, E. Z.; PLOTKIN, F. H.; FEIL, G. H.; WINKLER, D.; MARIK, S., and MARGOLIS, N.: Active physical reconditioning of coronary patients. *Circulation*, 32:110-111, 1965.
31. WHITE: *op. cit.*
32. CURETON: *op. cit.*
33. ECKSTEIN, R. W.: Effect of exercise and coronary artery narrowing on coronary collateral circulation. *Circ. Res.*, 5:230-235, 1957.
34. MOREHOUSE and MILLER: *op. cit.*
35. RUDD, J. L.: Cervical spondylosis: case report. *J. Amer. Geriat. Soc.*, 13:261-269, 1965.
36. KLUMPP, T. G.: Control of fatigue in the aging. *Virginia Med. J.*, 53:253-255, 1967.
37. MITCHELL, C.: New cure for sick hearts. *True The Man's Magazine*, 19:66-70, 1962.
38. RAAB, W.: Metabolic protection and reconditioning of the heart muscle through habitual physical exercise. *Ann. Intern. Med.*, 53:87-105, 1960.
39. TAYLOR, H. L.: The mortality and morbidity of coronary heart disease in men in sedentary and physically active occupations. *Amer. J. Public Health*, 52:697-707, 1962.

40. WHITE, P. D., and RUSK, L. W.: *Rehabilitation of the Cardiovascular Patient.* New York, McGraw, 1958.

41. GOLDSTEIN, M. S.; MULLICK, V.; HUDDLESTUN, B., and LEVINE, R.: The action of muscular work on transfer of sugars across cell barriers: comparison with the action of insulin. *Amer. J. Physiol.,* 173:212-216, 1953.

42. ENGERBRETSON, L.: The effects of exercise upon diabetic control. *J. Ass. Phys. Ment. Rehab.,* 3:74-78, 1965.

43. STEIN, J. U.: Motor function and physical fitness of the mentally retarded. *Rehab. Lit.,* 8:230-241, 1963.

44. OZARIN, L. D.: Corrective therapy in a psychiatric hospital. *J. Ass. Phys. Ment. Rehab.,* 8:3-4, 1958.

45. DAVIS, J. E.: *Rehabilitation: Its Principles and Practice.* New York, A. S. Barnes, 1946.

46. RUDD, J. L., and MARGOLIN, R. J.: The therapeutic value of the punching bag in physical and mental rehabilitation. *J. Ass. Phys. Ment. Rehab.,* 7:17-25, 1951.

47. ROSENBERG, D., and RICE, D. C.: Physical fitness and psychiatric diagnosis. *J. Ass. Phys. Ment. Rehab.,* 3:73-75, 1964.

48. JENKINS, R. L.: The role of the corrective therapist in the total phychiatric approach. *J. Ass. Phys. Ment. Rehab.,* 1:23-28, 1965.

49. JURICISIN, G., and HOWARD, A.: Persistence as a motivator. *J. Ass. Phys. Ment. Rehab.,* 1:16-24, 1964.

50. DENING, K.: Development of a corrective therapy program for the NB-TB patient at Brockton. *J. Ass. Phys. Ment. Rehab.,* 6:183-185, 1955.

Chapter IV

SOCIAL FACTORS IN MAINTENANCE THERAPY AND LONGEVITY

CHARLES L. ROSE

SOCIAL FACTORS has been conceptualized in this chapter to include broad sociological events, social change as epitomized by recent social welfare development, and the social-psychological matrix within which the patient is treated. Also, since maintenance therapy is essentially a life-prolonging procedure, the writer has taken this opportunity to sketch some of his own research on the social correlates of longevity. The research suggests predictors of the effectiveness of maintenance therapy and intervention to increase its effectiveness.

The concept of maintenance therapy has already been presented in previous chapters. It would not be amiss, however, to present a definition of maintenance therapy as it is related to social factors.

DEFINITION

There appear to be three essential ingredients in the concept of maintenance therapy: prevention, a "non-time-limited" characteristic, and an interdisciplinary approach.

Prevention

Prevention can operate at many levels: at a primary level where the condition is completely prevented from appearing in the first place; and at any one of later levels where the condition has already been established, but further worsening is prevented by specific procedures. Maintenance therapy is not concerned with the primary preventative level but rather with subsequent levels. When primary prevention fails or does not operate, diagnosis and treatment are instituted. These procedures may bring about a cure. However, if the condition is not cured and becomes chronic, then maintenance therapy would apply in order to prevent the condition from worsening. Thus, maintenance therapy can achieve a static condition by preventing further regression or may only succeed in decelerating the deteriorative process.

When the advance of the physical deteriorative process is affected, maintenance therapy may serve to maintain morale and thus achieve an improvement in the status of the patient. When treatment and rehabilitation have brought about an improvement, maintenance therapeutic procedures may be instituted in order to maintain improvement. Such procedures may also prevent recurrences or exacerbations. The significance of this aspect of maintenance therapy in the social area is that decrements in social functioning attendant upon chronic deterioration are cut down, and the pool of completely helpless individuals in the population is thereby lessened. Relative health is maintained for longer periods, and there is a general upgrading of the longevity characteristics of the population.

Non-time-limited Characteristic

The second aspect of maintenance therapy is its non-time-limited nature. Most therapies are time-limited and may either be of short-term or long-term duration. In maintenance therapy, however, there are no definitive time limits involved in the treatment. Maintenance therapy is applied for as long as it is needed to maintain the patient, and this of course may be for quite an indefinite length of time.

The maintenance concept is quite different from that involved in the theory of crisis intervention as propounded by Erich Lindemann and Gerald Caplan. The theory was originally developed for psychological and social types of intervention but can also be applied to medical intervention. The rationale is that mobilization of treatment at crisis points is more effective than at other times. With intervention occurring at the time of greatest need, the patient would conceivably then proceed on his own until the next crisis occurred. Having learned something from his experience with therapy during one period of crisis, the patient may not perceive the next crisis as quite so severe. Maintenance therapy, on the other hand, holds that there are large classes of situations in which maintenance is necessary between crises. Thus, the concepts of crisis intervention and maintenance therapy supplement each other and together succeed in covering all the possible situations which may occur.

The indefinite duration of maintenance therapy does raise some problems in the field of social policy with respect to the disposition of available means and manpower in the health care of the populace. Certainly the development of maintenance therapy would require an augmentation of trained personnel. As already stated, maintenance therapy has a preventative aspect and in this sense may have the effect of reducing the amount of over-all intervention necessary. Even with this effect, it is likely that in the end, more means and manpower would be needed. People who would otherwise die would be successfully maintained for longer periods, thus tying up an increment of medical means and personnel.

Interdisciplinary Approach

The third aspect of maintenance therapy is its interdisciplinary nature. It is not merely interdisciplinary within the medical and allied specialties but also within the social sciences. Social science interventions include the mobilization of personal influence techniques upon the patient as well as the restructuring of society, including subgroupings with the society, in order to make possible a general maintenance therapy program. Further illustrations of these points follow.

SOCIOLOGICAL ASPECTS
Demographic Shift

The first general sociological area to be considered is the ongoing demographic shift toward an increase in older age groupings in the population. Its relevance to maintenance therapy becomes apparent when one considers that older individuals are more prone to chronic conditions with which maintenance therapy tends to be associated. First, if a disease contracted in one's earlier years becomes chronic, then the residuals become more salient as one gets older. This occurs because with age an individual has less recuperative powers and has less capacity to deal with such residuals. Secondly, diseases of the senium tend to have a more chronic character, and so the older person is selectively a candidate for maintenance therapy.

Because of shifts toward greater longevity, there are greatly increased numbers of older people in the population. For example, the number of individuals aged sixty-five and over has increased from three million in 1910 to eighteen million in 1965, and it is expected that by 1970 this group will increase to twenty-five million. In addition, within the older age group from sixty-five and up there is a greater percentage increase in the older decades. For example, during the forty-year period from 1920 to 1960, there was almost a tenfold increase in the group aged eighty-five and over. Thus, older age population groups now exist which never before existed in any substantial numbers. Consequently, the need for maintenance therapy will become greater as time goes on.

The impression should not be left that maintenance therapy is utilized exclusively in the domain of the older age group; it also operates validly within younger patient groups. However, by comparison, the older groups are more prone to chronic conditions for which maintenance therapy is particularly suitable.

Attitudes

⎰The increase of aged groups in the population will bring about more positive attitudes toward them. The shift in attitude will, in turn, alter the position taken toward maintenance therapy for the aged. In a primitive society in which the aged were all but nonexistent, the older individual tended to be revered since he was a *rara avis*. The older individual tended to have a position of power and had control over material goods, and he was sought for advice and counsel. In a later period, when the numbers of the aged increased because of improvements in public health, sanitation, and advances in medical science, the older individual was less of an exception. The demands of an industrial society made his skills and talents less needed, and in the social upheavals which occurred in the transition from the agrarian to the industrial society, his care and maintenance was felt to be a burden. During this period, society became more youth-oriented, and the reverent attitudes toward the aged deteriorated. Although still in the throes of this stage, a third stage is beginning to emerge in which the aged are becoming more plentiful at a rapid rate. The means to support them have increased because of technological breakthroughs, and for these reasons, social attitudes toward them are becoming more favorable.

The trend to more favorable attitudes toward the aged is already betokened by the special provisions which have been enacted as part of the drive to the Great Society. The two landmark bits of legislation enacted in 1965 bearing on this point are Title XVIII of Public Law 89-97, the Medicare provisions of the Social Security Amendments of 1965; and Public Law 89-73, the Older Americans' Act of 1965. The emergence of changing attitudes toward the aged as related to their greater incidence in the population is manifested by a wealth of new social welfare provisions. These provisions will be discussed in a subsequent section.

Shift in Occupational Structure

Just as social and medical technology have brought about attitudinal and demographic shifts in the population toward the older age spectrum, industrial technology has brought about changes in the occupational structure. The general shift has been from manual to nonmanual occupations and has given greater importance to maintenance therapy for the group in the nonmanual occupational pool. Even with maintenance therapy, the physical demands of manual occupations would tend to make the objective of vocational rehabilitation more difficult to realize. On the other hand, when an individual in a non-manual occupation has developed a chronic condition, maintenance therapy would be more effective in maintaining his occupational role.

Two cases, that of carpenter and clerk, both of whom develop a disabling form of arthritis, will serve to illustrate. Maintenance treatment of the carpenter, even if effective, may not be sufficient to reduce his disability to the extent that he can go back to his work. On the other hand, even though a certain level of disability has already occurred, the clerk may still be able to go back to his work if, with maintenance therapy, his condition does not grow any worse. Also, even within the range of manual occupations, there has been, because of technological change, a shift to less physically arduous forms of manual work. Maintenance therapy would have a better chance to maintain an individual in his manual occupational role if he were a machine operator rather than a laborer.

Lowered Retirement Age

Another consequence of technological change relevant to maintenance therapy is the trend toward lowered age at retirement. Because of the primacy of the occupational role in our value system, the loss of this role creates problems for the individual despite programs of preretirement counselling and the development of postretirement leisure-time activities. When this problem in social adjustment is superimposed upon the development of a chronic condition, the management of the condition becomes more problematic.

Lowered morale in older age is known to be associated with poor physical health. Postretirement males are more apt to report lower morale if they have health problems than if they do not. Thus, as people retire at a younger age, they will be more vulnerable to this effect when they develop health problems. Thus, it becomes more important to institute widespread programs of maintenance therapy. As maintenance therapy arrests deterioration, it should decrease complaints regarding poor health and thereby lessen the loss of morale.

SOCIAL WELFARE ASPECTS

As part of the current war on poverty and the institution of the Great Society, there has occurred a revolution in social welfare. Three aspects of this revolution which are particularly relevant to maintenance therapy are the provisions of rehabilitation in public assistance, Medicare, and the Older Americans' Act. These three areas are consonant with and extend programs of maintenance therapy.

Public Assistance

In the public assistance category of Old Age Assistance, the 1962 Public Welfare Amendments provided for a program of social services to those in danger of becoming applicants for old age assistance. Study of old age assistance applications revealed that the major source of breakdown leading to dependency was the economic drain due to chronic illness. The provision in the 1962 Amendments to prevent such breakdown was to an important extent related to doing something about the depredations of chronic illness. By providing for this sort of preventative program, the demoralizing consequences of dependency could be averted or reduced. To accomplish this end was to prevent the ravages of chronic illness. An obvious approach was maintenance therapy by which an individual would be prevented from becoming more disabled; the greater disability which would impair earning capacity or at least the ability for self-maintenance would be averted. Maintenance therapy would also stave off the additional economic burden of increased medical expenses caused by the development of more serious medical conditions.

A second area in public assistance relevant to maintenance therapy was the Medical Assistance to the Aged program enacted in 1960. Under this program an individual would be eligible for aid if he were medically needy even though he might not be eligible to receive Old Age Assistance. An aged individual, then, would not have to wait until he became completely depleted before he could seek assistance. Thus, medical problems could be attended to before chronic deterioration became advanced. Medical Assistance to the Aged, therefore, encouraged the utilization of maintenance therapy. Social workers and re-habilitation workers who were harassed by the problem of finding resources for their clients have in Medical Assistance to the Aged a definitive resource for instituting maintenance therapy. This resource has been extended to other age groups by Title XIX of the Social Security Amendments of 1965, Public Law 89-97.

Another public assistance category calling for the use of maintenance therapy procedures is Aid to the Permanently and Totally Disabled. This program relates to the noninstitutionalized individual as do Old Age Assistance and Medical Assistance to the Aged. Its concern is with keeping noninstitutionalized people out of institutions by striving to prevent chronic illness from reaching the point at which institutionalization or hospitalization becomes necessary. The program specifically provides for reha-bilitation services in addition to public assistance, although its targets are the end products such as are involved in the permanently and totally disabled. Although it operates at this later level of "prevention," it still provides the opportunity through maintenance therapy of preventing even further deterio-ration and regression. The inclusion of younger groups from age eighteen onward, on the other hand, makes it possible to operate at an earlier level.

The most recent assist to maintenance therapy in the public assistance field is in Title XIX of Public Law 89-97, popularly known as Medicaid. This title extends the principle of medical assistance from the aged needy to needy of all ages. Under Title XIX it is not necessary for an individual to be permanently and totally disabled. In general, this title propounds, as does Medical Assistance to the Aged, that in order to be medically needy one does not first have to be on public assistance. For example, even a child who comes from a family in which the father is working but in which the income is inadequate to provide medical care may be eligible to receive medical benefits. Through such provisions the prevention of chronic illness in larger segments of the population is made possible. In fact, Medicaid is so broad that it potentially covers substantial numbers of the population under sixty-five and may even outstrip Medicare in scope.

Health Insurance

The second social welfare area highly relevant for maintenance therapy is Medicare, the popular designation of Title XVIII of Public Law 89-97. Since this area is dealt with in Chapter XII, treatment here will be very brief. Medicare is essentially health insurance for the elderly. Before the relevance of Medicare for maintenance therapy is set forth, the particular needs of the elderly for health insurance will be presented.

Briefly, the aged are more vulnerable to medical problems and the costs of medical care for two reasons: First, they are less capable financially than younger people; and secondly, they tend to be in poorer health. Their diminished financial capability with age, of course, is due to the loss of occupational role. For example, the median income of single, aged people including widowed individuals is about $1,000 per annum, while the median income of elderly couples is about $2,900 per annum. Also, after age sixty-five the percentage who must go on public relief rises. In the sixty-five- to sixty-nine-year age group, 6 per cent are on relief; in the seventy- to seventy-four-year age group, the percentage on relief rises to 11. For the next five-year age period, the rise is further to 18 per cent. For those over eighty, the percentage exceeds 25. The poorer health condition of the aged is documented by the National Health Survey: about 8 per cent of all those under age sixty-five suffer from disabling chronic conditions, while for those age sixty-five and over the figure rises to 40 per cent. Elderly people who tend to live on fixed incomes are further differentially victimized by inflationary medical costs. For example, from the period 1946 to 1961, during which time the consumer price index rose 53 per cent, medical costs went up 83 per cent. In view of these findings it was entirely rational for the benefits of health insurance to be given initially and preferentially to the aged.

Although Medicare is not a comprehensive scheme of health insurance for the aged, it does provide for hospitalization, nursing home care (extended care facilities), and visiting nurse care (home health services) as well as some outpatient care. Since the medical conditions of older people particularly require maintenance therapy, what Medicare essentially opens up, on quite a wholesale basis, is the expansion of maintenance therapy for older people.

Medicare is designed to assure a continuity of medical care, a circumstance which encourages the utilization of maintenance therapy. For example, in order to insure proper diagnosis and treatment, it is required under Medicare that before nursing home facilities are extended, the individual be hospitalized. Also, it is provided in this connection that there not be an extended hiatus between hospital discharge and entry into a nursing home. A further safeguard for continuity may be found in the provision that hospitalization and subsequent care in a nursing home be for the same illness. Furthermore, it is required that no longer than two weeks elapse between discharge from hospital or nursing home and the inception of the visiting nurse services.

Billions of dollars will be available to defray medical expenses of the elderly, paid for by payroll taxes and general revenues of the Federal Government. The potentials for increasing maintenance therapy programs are little short of astronomical. A tremendous amount of planning and research, therefore, is in order at this time to implement maintenance therapy.

The development of maintenance therapy has to date been blocked, in part at least, by a value system which favors acute treatment over long-term treatment for the chronically ill. Many more aged now exist, and tremendous new social welfare provisions have been made available for them. However, there is in the meantime a definite cultural lag in values which retards development of maintenance therapy. Inevitably, however, under the impact of demographic and legislative forces, the value system will change, as it is already beginning to change. The practice and development of maintenance therapy will be socially valued and esteemed as it has not been before. These value changes will reside both in the recipients of maintenance therapy, in the givers of maintenance therapy, and in the general population. As a result of this consensus, it will be natural and acceptable to focus on maintenance therapy rather than on acute treatment at the expense of maintenance therapy.

It may be predicted that eventually comprehensive health provisions for all segments of the population will be made available, possibly utilizing both the assistance and insurance principles. The result of such an eventuality may well be a general upgrading of the health of the general population. When this is coupled with expected breakthroughs in the conquest of disease—and specifically one thinks of the new Federal program on the conquest of the three major killers: cancer, heart disease and stroke—it may be anticipated that the need for maintenance therapy will eventually be obviated simply because diseases will be prevented from occurring in the first place or their effects will be nipped in the bud at an early stage. At the present time, however, even with fast-moving progress in the area of disease prevention, the concept of maintenance therapy is still a growing one, not an obsolete one. All, however, look forward with fervor to the time at which maintenance therapy will be obsolete.

Provisions for Older Americans

The third major development in the current social welfare revolution is an over-all program for the aged as epitomized by the Older Americans' Act of 1965. The act sets up under the Department of Health, Education, and Welfare a separate Aging Administration, a full-fledged sister of other administrations such as the Welfare Administration, the Vocational Rehabilitation Administration, and the Social Security Administration. As already stated, older age groupings are increasing rapidly, and they require special provisions and protection.

The problem of health maintenance in the aged is not unrelated to other areas of concern for the aged. Such other areas as expressed in the statement of objectives in the Older Americans' Act, in addition to attainment of physical and mental health, are as follows: adequate income; suitable housing; restorative institutional treatment; employment without discrimination due to age; a healthy, honorable, and dignified retirement; civic, cultural, and recreational opportunities; the preservation of freedom, independence, and individual initiative; efficient community services and social assistance; and the assurance of giving the aged the immediate benefit from research findings. Social, economic, cultural, and psychological provisions obviously assist in maintenance of the physical and mental health of the older individual. To achieve these objectives the Administration on Aging will act as a clearinghouse of information, assist states to develop special programs, administer special grants, develop research and demonstrations, keep statistics, publish educational material, and stimulate more effective use of resources already available in the community.

The Older Americans' Act is just the beginning of a concerted attack on the problems of the aged; the program will certainly grow in the years to come. All this will feed into the strengthening of the maintenance therapy concept for the older individual. Special programs for the aged already underway and to be greatly amplified are social group work, recreation, adult education, multiservice centers, "meals on wheels," protective services, special housing, employment, and preparation for retirement.

Although comparisons are odious, it is true, nevertheless, that there are other countries in the world who are ahead of the United States in provisions for the aged. One can think, for example, of the Scandinavian countries. There is no question that just as the United States is catching up in space research and emerging as the foremost country in this field, the United States will surely catch up and surpass all other countries (forgive the ethnocentrism) in provisions for the health and related types of care for the older citizen. The country is on the brink of vast social changes epitomized by the Great Society concept. The economy is providing the surpluses which are needed to develop these programs. The development of maintenance therapy will certainly play a significant part in this revolution.

The Poverty Problem

During a time of unparalleled prosperity in this country, there has been, paradoxically, a tremendous interest in eradicating poverty. Its relevance to maintenance therapy becomes apparent when one considers the well-known relationship between poverty and disability. For example, a study by the Department of Health, Education, and Welfare in 1963 showed that the incidence of heart disease in families of under $2,000 per annum income was five times that in families of over $7,000 per annum income. In the field of visual impairment there were nine times as many cases in the poorer families than in families with higher income. Furthermore, 87 per cent of the richer families possessed private health insurance while only one third of the poorer families had this kind of protection. In addition, the coverage was far less adequate for those poor families who carried insurance than for the better-off families who carried insurance.

The poor, therefore, are found to be more vulnerable to the costs of illness, have less protection from the costs of illness through insurance, and as a result become even poorer. Poorer groups are also less educated and are less apt to take advantage of the latest advances in medical knowledge, both because of lack of knowledge of available treatment facilities, and a reduced motivation to maintain health. A tendency exists, therefore, for chronic illness to develop more among the poor than among the middle and upper social classes and for maintenance therapy to be required more by the poor in a statistical sense.

Since maintenance therapy is concerned with the poor, it is important to assess the incidence and characteristics of poverty. A crude estimate of poverty in this country is that one fifth of the population is poor, comprising about thirty-five-million people. The poverty line for a nonfarm family of four is considered to be about $3,000 per annum, and since farmers receive part of their food and most of their housing without cash, the poverty line for the farm family is considered to require 40 per cent less cash income. About one-seventh of the poor either have no family or reside apart from their family. According to a 1963 census report, 35 per cent of poor families were aged, and 26 per cent were of broken homes with a female household head. Twenty-three per cent were nonwhite. With respect to educational level, 61 per cent of the adults in poor families had no more than an elementary school education. Eleven million of the poor are illiterate. Over 25 per cent are on public relief. These are the social characteristics of the groups in which chronic illness and the need for maintenance therapy tend to be concentrated. Successful application of maintenance therapy must take into consideration such patient characteristics, and special educational and motivational techniques should be employed in order that the cooperation of such groups might be gained.

It has become increasingly apparent in the antipoverty program that in order to gain the desired effect in reduction of poverty, the culture of the poor must be recognized. Those in the helping professions, be they social workers, rehabilitation workers, or physicians, tend to function as part of a higher socioeconomic level, and as a result tend to have less understanding of the culture of the poor. Problems in communication and rapport are thus created.

For example, the desirability for maintaining health may not be as much a part of the culture of the poor as it is a part of the middle-class culture. With respect to implementing maintenance therapy, the existing norms of the poor cannot be accepted but will have to be modified. In addition, special problems involving the aged, the Negro, the broken home, and poor education will have to be recognized in the construction of any large-scale maintenance therapy programs. However, in work with the poor, the proponents of maintenance therapy have an advantage in the already active and ongoing antipoverty program.

SOCIAL ASPECTS OF TREATMENT

The broader social aspects of maintenance therapy have specific implications for the social and psychological techniques necessary in the individual treatment situation. It is a truism that in addition to the medical and technical procedures involved in treatment one must carefully consider patient-therapist relationships and the social and cultural characteristics of the patient. All groups who work with patients should have this social orientation. The treatment situation involves working with the family to gain its cooperation in maintaining the level of improvement of the patient through the therapy period. The employment area is also involved, either in return to the job, retraining for another job, or in finding a job for the patient.

Community-centered Treatment

Because of the requirements of prevention and medical economics, treatment has shifted away from the intramural situation. In a community setting, be it an outpatient clinic, a social casework agency, or a rehabilitation workshop, the situation is less controlled than in a hospital or institutional setting. The many social forces operating on the patient must become part of the treatment plan. The remedy becomes more complicated but in the end is more realistic and comprehensive than in the intramural situation in which the patient is dealt with apart from the community from which he comes and to which he returns.

The shift into the community, the "natural habitat" of the patient, is illustrated in the psychiatric field by the tremendous growth of day-care centers and community mental health centers, and in the medical field by an increase in outpatient facilities and home care. The latter refers to teams of doctors and nurses going into the patient's home, as in the prototype program of the Montefiore Hospital and the better-established and older systems of visiting nurse care. In this context the burgeoning field of the nursing home may be viewed as an intermediary facility between the hospital and the community.

The Sick Role

Essentially, improvement of social functioning in the maintenance therapy patient entails the modification of the sick role in favor of the assumption of other roles, be they former roles or new roles. The sick role is legitimated by society on condition that the patient try to get well. The sick role is thus classically perceived as a temporary one. In this light, the chronic situation does offer some difficulties. The patient in this case does not get well quickly, and he tends to lose his motivation for getting well and for regaining his old social roles, such as that of work, because of the realities of his long-term illness. It is, therefore, very important for the maintenance therapist to prevent such social-psychological complications of chronic illness and to at least arrest its deteriorative effects.

At the same time a new way of life must be taught within the limitations of the *status quo* which has been achieved. The patient must be able to maintain a modicum of social functioning involving family roles, friendship roles, and even a modified form of work role or surrogate work role where the work role per se is contraindicated. The treatment emphasis is not so much on his illness but on his ability to function within the limitations of his illness. Involved is fragmentation of the sick role which will earn for the patient greater social approbation.

In summary, maintenance therapy is destined to assume a much greater importance in health care because of the far-reaching social changes currently going on in our society. Imperatives operating now which did not operate before are to conserve and maintain health. The economic, technical, and administrative means to realize this goal are being developed. Maintenance therapy will turn out to be no less esteemed than acute treatment. If a hierarchy of values remains, it will be treatment and prevention, with prevention in the superior position. The shift of health care out of the hospital into the community will simplify the problem of maintenance therapy because the patient will be dealt with in closer proximity to the social network of which he is a part. Dealing more fully with the social aspects of treatment, of course, makes the problem more complex, but in the end the objective of preventing chronic deterioration will be more effectively accomplished.

SOCIAL FACTORS IN LONGEVITY

In the last analysis, maintenance therapy is addressed to maintaining health and therefore to increasing longevity. It is thus germane to consider what social factors are associated with longevity. Such knowledge will identify those factors which in concert with maintenance therapy contribute to a longer life. Once these factors have been identified, they may be manipulated to supplement the longevity-increasing effects of maintenance therapy. Furthermore, the identification of those factors which are not manipulatable can at least serve as predictors of longevity, either positive or negative. Such social predictors could then indicate the effectiveness of maintenance therapy in prolonging life. In any case, knowledge of the social correlates of longevity is useful in a comprehensive approach to maintenance therapy.

Unfortunately, however, the state of knowledge regarding human longevity is extremely limited for three basic reasons: first, the prolonged human lifespan is discouraging to an investigator in that he cannot count on outliving his subjects and finishing his research; second, the interdiction of experimental control of the human; and third, the multivariate determinancy of longevity. Fortunately, information is available from insurance actuaries, based on experience with deceased life insurance policy holders and from death registration statistics gathered by the National Office of Vital Statistics. These sources offer two basic bits of information: a relationship between longer life and higher socioeconomic status, and a relationship between longer life and marriage. This suggests that maintenance therapy is more effective with those of higher socioeconomic status and with those who have the supportive advantage of married life. Further suggested is that the improvement of socioeconomic conditions and strengthening of family life is integrally related to building a program of maintenance therapy.

The author has conducted two studies to extend knowledge in this area: In the first study, the social characteristics of a group of long-lived males, Spanish-American War veterans, were compared to corresponding demographic norms. Those characteristics in which the longevous subjects departed from the norms were hypothesized to be related to longevity. In the second study, the next of kin (survivor-informants) of recently deceased individuals, as obtained from death certificates, were interviewed for biographical information on the deceased. This technique yielded data which were analyzed in their relationship to age at death both by univariate and multivariate procedures. The findings of these two studies will be briefly presented.

Spanish-American War Veteran Study

The 149 veterans who attended the Geriatric Clinic at the Boston VA Outpatient Clinic had an average age of eighty-two at the time they were studied. Their parents tended to be more long-lived than would be expected from the average longevity of their generation, and the mothers tended to be more long-lived than the fathers. It is likely that both genetic and social factors were operating. Long-lived parents may transmit to their offspring a superior genetic endowment and at the same time create a more favorable environment by maintaining for a longer period the primary fostering influence.

A second finding was that the veterans tended to be among the older siblings when the number of siblings was six or more. One explanation might be that older siblings have a competitive advantage over younger ones and have more responsibility earlier. Early responsibility is likely to facilitate emotional maturation and formation of adaptive skills. Another interpretation is that older siblings accrue certain biological advantages, since they were born when the parents were younger. Both these findings should sensitize the maintenance therapist to the importance of early family history in assessing the future of their patients.

The third general finding was consistent with demographic and actuarial findings regarding the relationship between socioeconomic status and longevity. The Spanish-American War veterans had a higher intelligence, higher education, and higher level of occupation than obtained in the general population. Apparently, these factors, highly interrelated on the basis of statistical tests of significance, afford a selective advantage in survival. Higher intelligence predisposes to higher educational attainment which in turn predisposes to higher occupational status. Higher status, in turn, is associated with less occupational hazard, higher earnings, and more favorable nutrition, sanitation, housing, and associated conditions. Finally, this more favorable environment would be conducive to longer life.

A fourth finding was that the elderly veterans had a higher incidence of marriage as compared with population norms, and more were still living with a spouse in their elderly years. The latter circumstance could be attributed to a tendency to remarry when their spouse died and to marry younger women in the first place. The interpretation is that "with-spouse status" is more favorable to longevity because it provides physical and emotional support. This tells the maintenance therapist that the patient will possibly respond better to the life-prolonging effects of treatment if he has a spouse to take care of him.

A final finding was that these veterans tended to maintain their occupational role beyond age sixty-five. Evidence of a refusal to disengage became even more remarkable when no relationship was found between current income and age of complete cessation from work. This suggested that these elderly gentlemen kept their fingers in employment out of a desire to remain useful or creative rather than for economic gain. The lesson is that maintenance of an occupational role or a surrogate thereof into elderly years bolsters longevity, perhaps because it bolsters self-esteem and a feeling of usefulness: Here is another area of treatment or social intervention which could augment the effectiveness of the maintenance therapist.

Survivor-informant Study

Five hundred lives of males in the Boston area who died from age fifty and up of natural causes during 1964 were studied. The survivor-informants were mostly wives who were in a position to give detailed and reliable information. A basic limitation, however, was the fact that the longer-living subjects were born earlier, thus introducing a secular effect in the direction of lower socioeconomic indices for those who lived longer.

The inability of this study to confirm the socioeconomic correlates of longevity was rendered less disturbing by virtue of the fact that the socioeconomic relationship to longevity has already been moderately well established through death registration and life insurance statistics. The study showed a significant relationship with longevity of subject's mother, but there was no correlation between subject's longevity and that of his father. Corroborating the Spanish-American War Veteran Study, correlations were found with marital status and older age than wife. Those who lived longer had also been more active physically and mentally during their lifetime than others of their own age.

In the occupational area there was no relationship to longevity, however, whether the job was supervisory or nonsupervisory or whether the subject got along with his boss. For those who survived beyond sixty-five there was a relationship between longevity and retirement adjustment as rated on the following scale: poor, fair, good, and even better than while working. There was a negative correlation between longevity and occupational stress and hazard.

With respect to smoking and drinking habits, there was a marked negative correlation between longevity and smoking. but there was no correlation with drinking. One has the feeling that the lack of social sanctions against smoking and the enormous sanctions against drinking may account at the social level for the greater lethal effect of smoking. Personality factors such as not being the worrying type, not being easily aggravated, and conserving one's energy also were related to longevity. Curiously enough, individuals who were rated as being trusting did not do so well with respect to longevity. On the other hand, being impulsive, planning for the future, giving up easily, and looking on the dark side of things did not seem to make any difference with respect to longevity.

The above findings give one food for thought with respect to what may be the important variables in making for longer life and what one can do about them. Those involved in maintenance therapy would do well to assess the socioeconomic status of their patients, their family characteristics, and personality characteristics with respect to relevance for longevity, since such factors influence the longevity-inducing effects of maintenance therapy. The findings presented are of course not hard and fast or final, since the research in this field is in its beginning phases. The findings, however, do have value in guiding and sensitizing those involved in prolonging life, both with respect to assessing the potential for prolonging life and intervention to increase this potential in areas other than maintenance therapy. With respect to intervention, it should be noted that factors relevant to longevity are operating over the lifetime of the individual, not merely at a later life stage when maintenance therapy is being applied. It follows that maintenance therapy ideally should be linked with earlier life-prolonging interventionist programs.

The findings regarding smoking deserve special comment. They confirm the large-scale studies performed by the National Institutes of Health and the American Cancer Society. It is unfortunate that smoking, unlike drinking, does not have a marked effect on behavior particularly with respect to loss of control, since the sanctions against drinking and lack of sanctions against smoking are undoubtedly related to this special behavorial effect. The problem is to construct an adequate basis for sanctions against smoking where a basis for sanctions does not naturally occur.

In addition to the univariate type of analysis described above, data in the survivor-informant study were also subjected to a multivariate analysis, specifically, a multiple regression procedure which produces a prediction formula. In a ten-variable prediction formula, smoking accounted for as much of the variance as all the other variables put together. Worrying, for example, accounted for one sixth of the variance accounted for by smoking, while marital status and mother's longevity each accounted for a mere one twentieth of the variance accounted for by smoking. Thus, multivariate analysis fully corroborated the univariate analysis used in the large-scale studies linking tobacco and mortality. It would follow that life-prolonging programs of maintenance therapy must be linked with programs of reduction in tobacco consumption earlier in the life of the individual. Unfortunately, this is not an easy matter, since there is further evidence from the multivariate analysis that smoking does not simply act as an independent variable but is in turn an outcome of other independent variables in the life style and personality areas, and in fact sums up these other variables which may be causally linked to longevity. The problem, therefore, is to prevent the development of certain traits and life styles (or to change them once they've developed) which result both in increased smoking and decreased longevity. This sort of preventative program is the sort of "preventative maintenance" which we have developed more enthusiastically for automobiles than for mere humans.

Maintenance therapy prolongs life just one little bit. Other factors prolong life, too, and all should be used together. It has been said that even if heart disease and cancer were conquered, the average expectation of life would rise only from seventy to seventy-five years, since there is a basic genetic limitation to longevity characteristic of the species *Homo sapiens.* Maintenance therapy, together with other procedures, should certainly play its part in maximizing years of life, the greatest gift of all.

Chapter V

MOTIVATION AND DEPENDENCY FACTORS

GEORGE J. GOLDIN

THE TERM *maintenance therapy, by* definition, implies maintenance of the physical, social, and emotional *status quo* against strong processes of deterioration due to aging and physical and emotional pathology and, as such, requires the utmost in motivation and resistance to dependency. It is the purpose of this chapter to analyze the positive and negative forces involved in motivating the patient and preventing inappropriate dependency. If the patient is to maintain his maximum level of functioning, he must be adequately motivated to participate actively in four major areas:

1. Strict adherence to the usually complex medical regimen.
2. Personal self-care functions for a modicum of independent living.
3. Rehabilitation exercises and related activities.
4. Psychosocial interaction with significant others in his social milieu.

In order that the patient be maximally motivated, the process of motivation must be conceptualized in its broadest sense. Barry and Malinovsky (1) have presented such a definition in the following statement:

> Motivation has been variously defined and described in terms of innate and learned drives and needs, in terms of inner stimuli and responses (both of which at times can be motivators), in terms of goals or the direction of motivation, and in terms of life values. One might say then that motivation concerns the extrinsic and intrinsic conditions responsible for variations in the intensity, quality, and direction of ongoing behavior.

These intrinsic and extrinsic factors are of crucial importance in conceptualizing the way in which the patient in maintenance therapy is motivated. This formulation means, in effect, that all psychosocial transactions in which the patient is engaged have a profound effect upon his motivation and his progress in maintenance therapy.

Similarly, Olshansky and Margolin (2) have described rehabilitation as taking place as a result of a dynamic interaction of social systems. Essentially, the geriatric patient in maintenance therapy has role partners (3) within three major social subsystems. These are the family, the community, and the medical subsystems, the latter of which in many cases is housed in a formal institution. When the patient is in a residential setting, a fourth subsystem, that of the institution itself, comes into play.

The influences and effects which these psychosocial transactions have upon the motivation of the patient will be analyzed in some depth. Family relationships and attitudes are major determinants of the patient's motivation to progress in successful maintenance therapy. Whether he is institutionalized or living at home, the feelings which family members mobilize in the patient either motivate him to strive to attain his highest level of functioning or indeed foster dependency and the eventual deterioration of his physical condition. For example, the family member who is overprotective of the patient stimulates anxieties concerning the patient's own condition and thus prevents his participation in exercise, daily living activities, and other rehabilitation procedures. On the other hand, family members who make demands on the patient for progress which is beyond his capacity evoke feelings of inadequacy which can depress the patient and serve as a block to his adequate maintenance in the therapy regimen.

If family members are pessimistic concerning the patient's condition, they very frequently communicate this pessimism when visiting the patient in any institutional setting and thus serve to impede his motivation in maintenance therapy. On the other hand, if they are overoptimistic to the point of being unrealistic, they build up the patient's hope for the attainment of levels which are impossible for him to achieve. If the patient being maintained is living at home, all the family conflicts and psychodynamic stresses which have been part of family living during the patient's life remain to throw him into conflict and produce emotional tension. Such tensions may not only have psychosomatic effects but can also serve to negate motivation and his efforts at trying to maintain himself at his current physical level.

It is vitally important for professionals who work with the patient in maintenance therapy to be highly cognizant of the effects of family dynamics upon the motivation of the patient. It is of profound value for doctors, nurses, social workers, physical and corrective therapists, and others who work with the patient to be able to interpret to the family the patient's physical problems. In this manner the family can conduct itself to function as an important motivating influence rather than a negative blocking factor. In other words, it is important for professional staff to counsel with families to assist in their acceptance of the patient's condition and to help them to help the patient maintain his physical *status quo* by adopting realistic but supportive attitudes.

Exactly which professional discipline carries on such counseling is not important. What *is* important is that the individual professional who is capable and who has a good relationship with the patient and his family undertake the counseling in an effort to improve the motivational climate which the family provides for the patient. In the past, it has been the social worker who has been allocated the role of counselor for families of patients. Although the medical social worker has specialized training in this area, members of other disciplines can carry it out quite satisfactorily if they understand something about the patient and the dynamics of family life.

Yet it must be remembered that some very sick geriatric patients who must be maintained in therapy have no families and live alone in the community. These patients who have arthritis, diabetes, and other complicated medical conditions require complex medical care involving a highly regulated treatment regimen which the patient must faithfully perform. Moreover, many of these geriatric patients suffer the emotional depression which comes with disengagement from their occupational and social roles. They feel inadequate, worthless, and useless. Feelings of rejection, of being unloved, unwanted, and unneeded take over. Patients in such an unmotivated condition become careless in following their treatment regimen and consciously and unconsciously reject it. Some even verbalize their own death wishes.

In these instances, the professionals in the medical, paramedical, and ancillary professions must occupy the role of substitute parents. Strong rapport must be developed, and their ability and willingness to help must be constantly and clearly communicated to the patient. The importance of community agency teamwork cannot be overemphasized. The home visit by members of home care teams such as the public health nurse and the social worker is crucial in the motivation of the home-bound geriatric patient. In addition, the community itself can be utilized to serve as a substitute for the family. In this regard, the social worker can be instrumental in mobilizing resources for the patient which are motivational in character—neighbors, social agencies, and recreational agencies. Such resource mobilization in the community requires that the patient's motivational needs be interpreted.

For the institutionalized patient in maintenance therapy, it might be necessary to counsel with families in order to motivate them to visit the patient and express love and concern. For others the goal might be to persuade the patient's family to visit less frequently because of their tendency to upset the patient. In any event the family must be recognized as a key factor in motivating patient participation in maintenance therapy.

Equally as important as the family is the professional staff which surrounds the patient. It is a truism that maintenance therapy cannot be carried on effectively without the cooperation of the patient. It might even be said that the progress of the patient is directly proportional to his motivation to participate in therapy. The acceptance of extensive medical schedules and complex medical procedures frequently requires that patients be motivated to work in partnership with medical personnel in order to arrest or retard the progress of physical pathology. Moreover, the patient must assimilate a strong commitment to the value of rehabilitation techniques. Such a commitment can only be inculcated by the professional staff with whom the patient comes in contact. Staff must be able to communicate a type of rehabilitation mindedness to the patient in order that he constantly strive to maintain and possibly increase his functional level. In institutional settings this rehabilitation mindedness must permeate and pervade the entire atmosphere.

Professional staff should allocate a portion of their time to talk with the patient and discuss his problems relative to the maintenance therapy regimen. This allows staff to encourage the patient, to individualize treatment, and in general, to give the patient the feeling that he is cared about by staff and that he is the concern of staff who *want* to help and what is more, *are* capable of helping. Such interpersonal relationships which exist between professional staff and the patient serve not only to clarify patient problems but also to give the staff member an opportunity to communicate confidence to the patient. This communication of confidence is a key factor in his motivation. If the patient can pick up a feeling of confidence about his condition from the staff, he will be far more motivated to continue to try to maintain himself on his current level of functioning.

Staff relationships with the patient as well as the relationship which exists among the staff members are of major importance to the patient's motivation. If there is a great deal of role conflict among staff members, and hostilities ensue, the tense atmosphere is quickly communicated to the patient. A natural consequence is an anxiety reaction on the part of the patient. Studies have repeatedly shown that staff conflict and tension affect the progress of patients in an institutional setting. Perhaps this was best demonstrated by Stanton and Schwartz (4) in their study of mental hospitals. While there is certainly room for honest differences of opinion among staff members concerning the care of patients and individual patients in particular, all staff members must be united in their commitment to a rehabilitation philosophy and to the value of maintenance therapy. If staff consensus does not exist in this area, then irresolvable tensions will exist and may have detrimental effects upon the motivation of the patient in maintenance therapy.

The importance of staff relationships to the patient evolves from the fact that the patient cloaks staff members in an aura of authority. This authority is perceived by the patient as the capacity for the medical and paramedical personnel to grant life and health. It is almost a magical-thinking type of investment. However, such perception of medical personnel by patients in maintenance therapy does exist and must be considered. This aura of authority can be used to great advantage by the staff in motivating the patient to try and to work hard in his maintenance therapy regimen.

The management of dependency in the maintenance therapy patient is a major problem for the professional staff in whose care he is assigned. The patient suffers most from a type of dependency which the author terms *psychomedical* (5). By psychomedical dependency is meant the reality-induced dependency which accrues from illness. Because of his incapacity, the patient is compelled to rely on others to satisfy his basic wants and needs. Such dependency is a particularly difficult problem for the patient in maintenance therapy because he knows very well that his illness is chronic and, as such, that he can never return to a state of full independence. Moreover, the maintenance therapy regimen itself requires that the patient be completely dependent on a number of individuals for his continued life and existence. This particular situation may never be openly clarified for the patient. However, he usually has a dimly conscious or at least preconscious awareness of his status.

The chronically ill patient usually responds to this position of forced dependence by one of two personality reactions. Some patients regress, becoming very childlike in their relationships with those whose role it is to care for them. This type of patient develops into a complaining, demanding individual who is totally dependent and almost incapable of any goal-directed behavior. His motivation is either at a low ebb or negative in character. The other response to psychomedical dependency takes the form of a denial reaction. In this response the patient lapses into such conflict over his dependent position that he refuses to accept this role and rejects the help of those about him.

Both reactions can pose serious problems for a staff charged with the responsibility of providing maintenance therapy to the chronically ill; yet a staff who understands the dynamics of dependency can motivate patients in the direction of cooperation and a meaningful life. There are definite procedures for coping with accentuated dependent behavior of patients in maintenance therapy. These procedures are as follows:

1. The staff and those whose role it is to provide the patient with care must first and foremost be able to accept the initial barrage of his dependent behavior. The staff member should be able to communicate to the patient that he understands the patient's dependent strivings and thinks none the less of him in spite of his dependent position. It is important that the staff and family of the patient clarify to him that dependency due to illness does not mean subservience or lowered esteem in their eyes.

2. The patient should be helped to feel that he has a measure of control over his destiny and what is being done to him and for him. It is important to remember that a chronically ill patient in maintenance therapy feels particularly vulnerable and helpless. In this regard he must be given the feeling that a certain measure of self-determination is his.

3. Although universalization is no solution to the patient's dependent situation, it does help to know that there are others in his position who have been helped to make adequate adjustments and live relatively happy lives. Some degree of universalization for the patient by the staff does help to instill a higher level of confidence and hope.

4. Doctors, nurses, social workers, and other professionals can enable the patient to realize that if he is faithful to maintenance therapy and rehabilitation procedures a certain amount of gratifying independent functioning is still possible for him. This can be communicated constantly and to some extent can be based on medical facts.

The term *rehabilitation* implies a combatting of dependency.

[This means, in effect, that any setting in which maintenance therapy is carried on must espouse and indeed be permeated by a rehabilitation philosophy or rehabilitation mindedness. This philosophy dictates that all activities of the particular setting be geared to helping the patient achieve his maximum potential for self-care and socially and psychologically constructive relationships.]

Unfortunately, such is not always the case. Indeed, in many institutional settings a type of institutional dependency (6) is fostered. It is not uncommon, where large numbers of patients are being treated, for activities to become highly routinized for the convenience of staff. In such settings, efforts of the better-motivated patient for independent actions are resisted and even frowned upon if such action disrupts the institution's operational patterns. For example, a patient in a nursing home may want to dress himself, but because of his slowness and the time it requires he is discouraged. Naturally, without encouragement such motivation for independent achievement soon becomes extinguished.

The very character of institutional life with its monotony, paucity of new experience, and its isolation from the reality of community life decreases positive motivation and increases dependency. Usually the patient is sheltered, overprotected, and knows that his basic material wants will be met whether or not he initiates any independent activity. Such knowledge very frequently blocks the patient's independent strivings to do things for himself.

It is common knowledge that all human beings have certain emotional and social needs which must be met if they are to be well motivated. Certainly the patient in maintenance therapy is no exception, and indeed the requirement for need-meeting is even more pronounced and important for the chronically ill patient.

Almost fifty years ago the sociologist W. I. Thomas (7) set down a group of four basic human psychosocial needs. Thomas maintained that only if these needs were satisfied could an individual make a healthy adjustment to life. These four needs are security, recognition, response, and new experience. Over the years this need model has been criticized on the basis that it is oversimplified and does not hold true in all situations. Nevertheless, in a general way it makes sense. An examination of these four needs clearly indicates their importance in motivating the patient in maintenance therapy and reducing his dependency.

The patient's need for security is certainly of paramount importance. As has been indicated earlier, the patient in maintenance therapy, as a chronically ill patient, feels exceedingly vulnerable. He is dependent on others for his very life. If he is to be motivated to try, he must feel secure in the knowledge that those about him will not let him down and that he can count on them for all types of support—medical, social, and emotional. The patient must feel that there will be a consistency of response from those about him which will enable him to predict their behavior in given situations so that he can pattern his reactions to the cues and stimuli of the significant others in his environment. It is important that as far as possible, those responsible for the maintenance therapy of the chronic patient give their actions a measure of predictability so that the anxiety of the patient will be reduced. This means that the staff and those about the patient should act the same way in particular situations over a period of time and also do their best to prepare the patient for any new experiences or procedures which will take place in his behalf. In other words, the patient must feel that all staff, family, and others with whom he comes in contact can be relied upon as people who are working for his own best interests.

Recognition is required by all human organisms and is vital to motivation. Whether it is for baking an apple pie, being a great statesman, or merely being pleasant to be with, every individual must feel that he is recognized for something, some special thing, related to himself. Without some special form of recognition, all individuals are open to the development of profound feelings of inadequacy.

For the patient in maintenance therapy, recognition is doubly important. Because his capacities have been drastically curtailed and his former abilities reduced, the chronically ill develops very strong feelings of inadequacy and inferiority. Because of these feelings, it is most important for the staff and family of the patient to look for instances in which they can give him recognition. Whether it is for achievements in occupational therapy, cooperation in treatment, or for relationships with other people in the institution, the patient must be recognized. Recognition, in effect, gives the patient a reason for being and motivates him to increase participation in his treatment plan.

Emotional response is a crucial factor in the motivation of the patient in maintenance therapy. By *emotional response* is meant the ability of people around the patient to communicate understanding and empathy. Perhaps the term *love* might be used synonymously with *response*. Coupled with and part of the response factor is the ability of the various medical and paramedical personnel as well as the patient's family to listen to the patient and his problems. By the term *listen* is meant to listen without barriers to communication. All too often people expose themselves to communicated information without ever really integrating it. For the patient in maintenance therapy, it is vitally important to pay careful attention to his problems, his complaints, his aspirations, and his desires. This does not mean that all his whims and vagaries must be gratified. However, it does mean that he must be attended to as an individual in need of help and his basic needs evaluated and responded to.

Finally, the patient's needs for new experiences must be met. New experiences serve as prime stimuli in motivating the patient in maintenance therapy. Because of the limitations of the patient as well as the limitations and boundaries of institutional life, it is not always simple to provide new experiences for the chronically ill. Nevertheless, with creative efforts of the staff it is possible to involve patients in activities which are new and enriching.

One of the ways in which this can be achieved is by linking the institution to the community. It is possible through the utilization of volunteers and outside contacts to bring the community into the institution and interpret the institution to the community. Such efforts usually result in a relationship between the two which facilitates new experiences for patients. For those living at home there is always the opportunity for bringing in new and stimulating people to talk with them as well as teach them new recreational and avocational skills.

Thus far, motivation and dependency of the patient in maintenance therapy as responses to a complex interplay of psychodynamic and sociodynamic forces have been discussed. However, they can also be viewed in their simplest form as operant responses to positive and negative reinforcement. Reward can take the form of praise; such praise by one in authority can go a long way in motivating the patient to try.

However, what must be remembered is that the geriatric patient is a potentially fragile person and that his motivating stimuli must come not from one or two persons but from a total milieu which is encouraging and therapeutic in character. Whether the patient resides in an institution, lives with his family, or lives alone, those with whom he comes in psychosocial contact must be supportive. In this regard the janitor of the building is as important as the most professionally trained clinician. It is the communicated general interest in the patient by everyone around him which motivates him, and it is the refusal of these same people to do things for him which he is able to do for himself which helps fight dependency.

Another area of major importance in considering the necessity for motivating the geriatric patient is the prevention of psychosomatic illness and the exacerbation of existing illness by psychological stress. One psychological problem in this realm is that of accident proneness. Those who work with the geriatric patient have noted that when he becomes depressed, anxious, or lacks motivation, he tends to have accidents which result in incapacitation and increases in demands for love and a dependent position.

Yet the importance of "tender loving care" (TLC) cannot be minimized. A recent study involving the motor performance of handicapped individuals (8) indicated that an accepting, warm attitude by the individual experimenter in a position of authority may have contributed to the overriding of monetary and status incentives as factors motivating subjects to try harder. The acceptance and warmth of the experimenter also negated status rewards as motivational factors.

Another study of dependency ongoing at the New England Rehabilitation Research Institute is predicated on the hypothesis that there is a relationship between the individual's inability to make decisions and his dependent strivings. If this hypothesis is substantiated, an entirely new counseling dimension will unfold. As decision-making-oriented counseling is carried on with the patient, his ability to make decisions might be improved and his independent function increased.

Finally, it is important to note the need for research in the area of motivation and dependency of the geriatric patient in maintenance therapy. The following are a number of questions upon which many opinions are expressed but for which there are no objective data:

1. What are the characteristics of the patient who is motivated best by professionals of a given sex?
2. What are some of the psychodynamic reasons for the patient's rejection of medication?
3. From a psychosocial standpoint, what type of patient does best living alone? in an institutional setting?
4. From the standpoint of operant conditioning studies, what schedules of reinforcement will most effectively motivate dependent patients?
5. What is the role of the volunteer in motivating the geriatric patient?
6. What effects does organizational structure have upon the capacity of staff to motivate patients?
7. What group dynamics techniques (role-playing, and so on) are most effective in motivating the geriatric patient?
8. Finally, in what ways do geriatric patients motivate each other? The idea of mutual help among individuals with problems is not new and is being increasingly explored in community action programs. In hospitals, such mutual motivation takes place spontaneously. However, such activity can be stimulated, utilized, and studied.

In summing up, the motivation of the geriatric patient in maintenance therapy is a "total pack" proposition based upon the patient's physical and emotional capacity. A dynamic approach is necessary because the patient is struggling to keep afloat in a society which is attempting to free itself from him. Most frequently this process of disengagement is spoken of as if it were unidirectional, that is, the elderly patient isolating himself from society and family. On the contrary, disengagement takes place not only when the patient segregates himself from the social group but when the social group isolates itself from the patient. This fact is substantiated by society's constant effort to segregate the elderly in the areas of housing, recreation, medical care, and so forth. The excuse frequently given is that the elderly are more comfortable with each other. There is little research to support the truth of this assertion; if, indeed, it is true, it does not necessarily follow that the patient benefits.

Segregation and disengagement frequently take place not as a result of the geriatric patient's own motivation but rather as a result of the motivation of those about him. Many times, guilt, overidentification, and fear of the aging serve as motivating forces for some individuals to disengage themselves from the elderly or to push the elderly towards disengagement.

The geriatric case mobilizes a variety of feelings in those who live and work with him. It must always be remembered that it is these feelings which serve to help or block maintenance of the elderly patient.

REFERENCES

1. Barry, J. R., and Malinovsky, M. R.: Client motivation for rehabilitation: a review. *Rehabilitation Research Monograph*, No. I, U. of Fla., 1965.
2. Olshansky, S., and Margolin, R. J.: Rehabilitation as a dynamic interaction of systems. *J. Rehab.*, 29:17-18, 1963.
3. Merton, R. K.: Reference groups and social structure. *In Social Theory and Social Structure.* New York, Free Press of Glencoe, Inc., 1957, pp. 368-379.
4. Stanton, A. H., and Schwartz, M. S.: *The Mental Hospital.* New York, Basic Books, 1954.
5. Goldin, G. J. and Perry, S. L., with the collaboration of Margolin, R. J. and Stotsky, B. A.: Dependency and its implications for rehabilitation. Northeastern Studies in Vocational Rehabili-

tation, 1967, No. 1. Boston, Massachusetts, Northeastern University.

6. *Ibid.*
7. Thomas, W. I.: *The Unadjusted Girl.* Boston, Little, 1923.
8. Perry, S. L., and Stotsky, B. A.: Type of reward, incentive, and incentive-sequence as factors in the motor performance of mentally retarded, physically handicapped, and college students. *J. Psychol., 60:*55-65, 1965.

Chapter VI

NUTRITIONAL MANAGEMENT OF GERIATRIC PATIENTS

MARIE M. ALEXANDER AND FREDERICK J. STARE

KNOWLEDGE and understanding of the nutritional needs of geriatric patients is a relatively recent development. Throughout history, man has speculated on the relation of foods to longevity, but only now, when longevity has become a reality, is there beginning to be enough data and experience to throw light on this subject.

Many questions come to mind as centenarians grow in number: Is there a combination of foods or nutrients which can slow down the process of aging? What is the relationship of dietary factors to chronic illness or pathological conditions? Is there a nutritional formula which can enhance life in the late decades?

Complete answers still lie in the future. Yet even today's knowledge assigns a big role to nutrition in the maintenance therapy of the elderly. Research on the connection between diet and cardiovascular disorders or diabetes and on the hazards of obesity provides convincing proof that nutrition is important in the prevention of disease. Studies also indicate that there is a high correlation between a balanced diet in early years and maintenance of vitality in later years. It becomes increasingly more evident that lifelong good food habits are excellent insurance against poor nutrition and its associated complications in old age.

Unfortunately, large segments of the general population do not practice good food habits. This is particularly true of the elderly, and with this group, multiple physiological, social, economic, and psychological factors create added complications.

109

Overeating, undereating, and misguided eating are characteristic of all too many of our aged.

There are important reasons for trying to correct this situation. Many conditions are complicated by poor nutrition. Symptoms such as weakness, tiredness, and lack of appetite often reflect subclinical nutritional deficiencies and respond well to correction. The dramatic improvement which results increases an individual's comfort and strength and in addition enhances his efficiency and sense of independence. The favorable psychological reaction derives both from the patient's greater feeling of vigor and also from his realization that there is something positive which he can do to help himself.

Without question, total rehabilitation is unattainable without nutritional rehabilitation. With good nutrition the individual is physically better equipped to perform at his particular maximum and emotionally better able to enjoy his added years.

The physician must be both doctor and counselor, trained to evaluate a patient's nutritional status, to be sensitive to environmental as well as medical problems, and to be able to encourage the patient to obtain foods which will satisfy his particular nutritional, social, and emotional requirements. Therefore, this chapter will cover normal nutritional needs for the elderly and also adjustments which are indicated in various disorders. Careful consideration will be given to environmental factors which influence the nutritional pattern. Finally, foods and plans will be suggested which can be beneficial to the patient, to the physician, and to others concerned with optimum nutrition for "the closing years."

NUTRITIONAL REQUIREMENTS

Fundamentally, the guiding principles of good nutrition are the same at eighty as at thirty: The daily food must be sufficient to supply all essential nutrients, and caloric intake must be regulated to accord with energy needs. The only difference is that in old age caloric reduction is usually greater and the achievement often harder than in middle age. Also, with some elderly individuals, it may be desirable to alter the meal pattern in order to permit frequent small feedings. However, whatever the distribution, the total should provide the following essentials.

Carbohydrate

Young and old alike derive about 40 to 50 per cent of their calories from carbohydrates. In management of the elderly, whose caloric intake is reduced, it is important that the carbohydrate not be supplied by a disproportionate amount of sweets; these have the double disadvantage of filling the patient only with calories and dulling the appetite for other foods. As total consumption declines, it is advisable to recommend carbohydrates which carry minerals and vitamins, such as enriched or whole grain bread and cereals, and fruits and vegetables.

Protein

The National Research Council recommends that the protein requirement of one gram per kilogram of body weight be maintained even with advancing age. Since total food consumption is diminished, a higher proportion of the total must come from protein. Often, fatigue, edema, and lowered resistance to infection are related to a low protein intake. In addition, hypoproteinemia is often associated with senile pruritis, bedsores, and poorly healing wounds.

Adequacy of protein requires balance between "complete" and "incomplete" proteins. Complete contain all the "essential" amino acids (those which cannot be synthesized by the body) and are supplied by food from animal sources (meat, fish, poultry, and dairy products). Incomplete come from grains and vegetables. The two complement each other, so a small amount of milk served with cereal, or a small portion of meat, fish, or poultry accompanying rice, potato, or spaghetti will make the total protein complete and nutritious.

Fat

Current opinion suggests that most adults would be wise to exercise moderation in total fat intake, to reduce their consumption of saturated fat and cholesterol, and to add some polyunsaturated fats to the daily diet. This is probably a good general principle to follow in outlining a nutritional regimen for the elderly.

Minerals

The mineral requirement does not decrease with increasing years, but surveys show that at least some of these essential nutrients are often slighted by elderly individuals.

Calcium

Calcium is frequently deficient. This is unfortunate, since an inadequate intake over a long period of time may be a factor in the development of osteoporosis. Though such longstanding neglect cannot be rectified, an adequate intake is definitely of importance to supply the requirements of bones and fluids.

Increasing calcium intake is frequently difficult to achieve because milk is avoided by many individuals who consider it "constipating" or gas-producing. Often in these cases skimmed milk or boiled milk or cheese are successful alternatives. Those who skimp on milk because of its cost can be introduced to evaporated milk. Dried skimmed milk is also a good substitute. It is low in cost, easy to store, and can be used not only as a beverage but also as a supplement with soups, cereals, or even with a glass of whole milk.

Iron

Although bodily needs for iron do not diminish with the years, the intake often drops. There are recent suggestions that iron intake is marginal. Because meat can be costly or difficult to prepare or chew, it is often excluded by the elderly. Therefore, it is advisable to stress the importance of meat, or a weekly serving of liver, and of other iron-rich foods such as egg yolk, dried beans and peas, dark green leafy vegetables, and whole grain or enriched breads and cereals.

Sodium

Sodium is a mineral which poses no problem unless the intake must be restricted. In this instance, maintenance therapy can be a challenge to the physician who must help the patient learn to make the necessary dietary modifications. Incidentally, the physician should be aware that when iodized salt is omitted, iodine insufficiency may develop as a concomitant of the sodium restriction.

Potassium

Potassium needs are fully met by a balanced diet, unless the patient is receiving a diuretic. This necessitates careful attention to the potassium-rich foods such as citrus fruits, cantaloupe, bananas, apricots, prunes, and vegetables.

Fluorine

The role of fluorine and the value of supplemental fluoride in the treatment or prevention of osteoporosis has still to be fully delineated. Nevertheless, an optimal intake of fluoride, through the use of fluoridated water, is as beneficial to the elderly as it is to everyone else.

Vitamins

With vitamins, as with minerals, needs of the elderly are unchanged, but intakes are often poor. When foods are not carefully chosen, the supply of vitamins is usually far from adequate, and vitamin C is often missing entirely. This may be due to a widespread tendency to classify fruit juices as "hard to digest, acid foods." Since fruits and juices which supply ascorbic acid are easily obtained, require no preparation, and need not cause digestive difficulties, the desirability of reeducation is obvious. Deficiency of other vitamins is also often a result of ignorance, so the challenge to the physician is clear.

As a matter of fact, he is faced with a two-pronged responsibility: He must give information about vitamin-rich foods and at the same time counteract the common misuse of vitamin supplements. A recent survey in Rochester, New York, underlines facts, familiar to many nutritionists, about the wastefulness of vitamin preparations. One half of the people interviewed who were buying vitamins already had good diets. Seventy-five per cent of the others were purchasing preparations which failed to supply the vitamin or vitamins lacking in their particular diet. The best way, even for the elderly, to obtain all the vitamins as well as all the other essential nutrients, is through careful selection of foods.

Calories

The goal for all adults is to maintain "desirable weight," the average weight for a given height and each sex at age twenty-five. To achieve this necessitates for many a gradual decrease in caloric intake, since with advancing years there is a progressive decrease both in activity and in bodily energy requirements.

As a general guideline, the National Research Council recommends that calorie allowance be reduced by 5 per cent per decade between the ages of thirty-five and fifty-five, by 8 per cent for ages fifty-five to seventy-five, and up to 10 per cent for those over seventy-five. This, of course, must be further adjusted if a patient is confined to bed or a wheelchair or is very inactive.

Those individuals are fortunate who have kept their calories in balance and have maintained a desirable weight. All others should be advised to regulate calories so that desirable weight is reached and maintained.

Water

No survey of normal requirements is complete without mention of water. Inadequate intake of liquids is characteristic of the elderly and a common cause of constipation. Older people need to be reminded to have six to seven glasses of fluid per day.

Fiber

Some fiber is also usually indicated to prevent or treat constipation. Frequently, individuals do not realize the value of cooked fruits and vegetables in this connection. Also, others need information to counter their queer notions about "roughage" and their preconceived, often stubborn, opinions about the desirability of avoiding certain fruits, vegetables, or grains.

A BASIC FOOD PLAN

The danger with many *elderly* persons is their tendency, for any one of many reasons, to restrict their food intake to a few food items. The aim, therefore, must be to stress the wisdom of variety in the choice of foods.

The ideal is to teach the patient about what is called the Basic Four. This is simply an easy guide to good nutrition. Anyone who conscientiously follows this outline will be most likely to receive an adequate supply of protein, minerals, vitamins, and the other essentials. Addition of fats and other foods should depend on caloric and nutrient requirements.

The Basic Four

Dairy Products

Every day the elderly individual should have one pint of milk or its equivalent for calcium, protein, and vitamins. This can be whole milk or skimmed milk, evaporated or dry milk, or buttermilk. One ounce of cheddar-type cheese or one-half pint of cottage cheese or of ice cream are approximate calcium equivalents of one glass of milk.

Vegetable-Fruit Group

Four daily servings of vegetables and fruits supply vitamins, minerals, and fiber. One serving should be citrus (for vitamin C), and at least four times a week the intake should include a dark green or deep yellow vegetable or fruit for vitamin A.

Meat Group

Two servings daily of meat or poultry or fish supply protein, iron, vitamins, and also fat. One serving should be dinner-sized (two or three ounces without bone or fat) and one should be lunch-sized (one egg or an ounce of cheese, meat, or fish). Two eggs or one cup of dried peas, beans, or lentils or four tablespoons of peanut butter are protein equivalents of a medium serving of meat. Cereal or bread with milk also provides protein.

Bread-Cereal Group

Four servings daily of enriched or whole grain breads and cereals supply carbohydrate, minerals, and vitamins. A serving is a slice of bread, three quarters of a cup of ready-to-eat cereal, or about one half of a cup of cooked cereal, cornmeal, grits, macaroni, noodles, rice, or spaghetti.

PHYSICAL CONDITIONS WHICH AFFECT REQUIREMENTS

Since the Basic Four provides a flexible pattern, it can serve as the framework within which any patient's daily intake can be achieved. Frequently, it must be altered to accommodate special individual situations. Following is a guide to some of the more common modifications which may need to be made for optimum maintenance therapy.

Lack of teeth or poorly fitting dentures may create nutritional problems. The physician has to be alert to the fact that the patient may be restricting his intake to a few soft foods unless he is instructed in making wiser adjustments. The patient also needs to be warned against overcooking to achieve tenderness, since this can destroy the taste and appeal of the food as well as some of its nutritive value.

Poor food habits or poor nutrition may also be a consequence of infection. They sometimes result too if a patient has difficulty in swallowing or if a decreased sense of smell causes loss of appetite. Other patients develop strange habits in attempts to treat constipation or "acid stomach" or "spastic bowel."

Physical defects may also affect nutritional status, though not necessarily altering nutritional needs. Even though an individual might know about good nutrition, such handicaps as poor vision, poor locomotion, general frailty, or difficulty in eating may have disastrous effects on the food intake. Outside of these various medical situations which may lead to poor nutrition, there are disorders which actually require dietary modifications.

Overweight and Underweight

At the International Association of Gerontology Meeting in Copenhagen, August 1963, it was stated that "a substantial number of elderly people are undernourished and about the same proportion are overnourished." Certainly, rectifying this situation is important in nutritional rehabilitation.

In all instances, of course, if there is an underlying pathology, it must be taken into consideration and be treated. For example, malnutrition may be secondary to infection or other disease. Obesity may be associated with diabetes, cariovascular disorders, or arthritis. Both underweight and overweight, however, usually reflect poor food habits and respond well if these are corrected.

Actually, since marked overweight decreases the life span, it is more common among the aging than among the aged. Even older adults, however, often pay a large penalty for surplus pounds. Overweight is an added complication in high blood pressure, diabetes, and cardiovascular disease. Moreover, obesity impedes locomotion, and this can aggravate arthritis. Excess weight may also complicate recovery from injury and from surgery.

Yet weight reduction, hard to achieve at any age, is especially difficult with older individuals. There are several psychological barriers which the physician must do his best to overcome if treatment is to be successful. Long accustomed to getting along with excess weight, individuals may not believe it is truly harmful. Entrenched in their own ways, they may stubbornly cling to their time-honored habits. Also, with some patients, food becomes a chief source of satisfaction, as other sources of gratification are limited, and the doctor may have to work hard to find some substitute.

Dietary restriction in this age group is further complicated by the fact that with advancing age, the lowered basal metabolic rate and reduced physical activity create a vicious circle. Because the patient needs less and moves less (especially when he suffers from arthritis or other physical handicaps), he tends to put on more weight, and then the added pounds simply reduce his activity and his caloric requirement still more.

Success in imposing a reducing regimen depends in large measure on the doctor's patience and powers of persuasion. A big hurdle is overcome if the patient can be convinced that weight loss will increase his independence and ameliorate some of his symptoms.

The diet itself should be fitted as closely as possible to the individual's habits, likes, dislikes, and living conditions as well as nutrient needs. The patient should be urged to divide the total caloric allowance into three regular meals and probably also into one or two extra snacks. Emphasis should be placed on exclusion of high-calorie items with concentrated sweets or fats. The physician must be specially cautious to make sure that when the patient is decreasing his total intake he does not at the same time decrease his intake of essential nutrients. The basic four foods must all be included to insure a sufficiency of protein, minerals, and vitamins. If the patient is taught to use a variety of foods and to cut *down*, rather than *out*, the hope is that he will gradually learn to eat well while he is eating less.

Frequently, adding calories is as difficult for the underweight person as eliminating them is for the overweight, and again, psychological factors complicate the picture. Sometimes, self-imposed food restriction is used to win attention or affection. It is helpful if the patient can be convinced that malnutrition may be aggravating his other symptoms, such as weakness, susceptibility to infection, or general irritability.

The best advice is to start with the Basic Four and then make gradual additions to the total daily intake, emphasizing the rich foods which contain concentrated calories. Meals should be regular and relaxed. Extras between meals are often desirable if taken when they do not dull the appetite for the next meal, and a substantial snack at bedtime is often helpful. Progress may be slow, but with such a regimen it should be steady.

At this time it is well to stress the desirability of even a little regular exercise. Unless this is physically impossible, moderate and appropriate physical activity is a highly desirable adjunct to good nutrition as well as to the treatment of overweight and underweight. By improving muscle tone, burning up extra calories in the overweight, stimulating appetite in the underweight, exercise makes an important contribution to nutritional rehabilitation and frequently provides a feeling of vigor, well-being, and accomplishment.

There are, of course, other pathological conditions in which dietary adjustments will be necessary. To accommodate dental or gastrointestinal situations, food texture may have to be altered. Diabetes may dictate a reduction in bread or cereal or fat. If sodium or potassium is a consideration, other changes may be indicated. A general discussion cannot be more specific, since in all these conditions diets must be precisely figured to meet individual requirements. However, whatever the condition, whenever possible the modifications should always include the foods in the Basic Four.

OTHER CONDITIONS WHICH AFFECT NUTRITION

Environmental as well as medical factors may profoundly affect a patient's nutritional status and determine his food practices. Awareness of these influences is basic to adequate nutritional rehabilitation.

Income, of course, is frequently a major consideration in the lives of the aged. It is well known that food often suffers if it must compete with other items in a tight budget. This may be aggravated when an elderly person is trying to manage on a greatly restricted retirement allowance. Often, however, this can be alleviated if the patient receives good counsel about planning and purchasing. Simple suggestions relating to wise economies and low-cost nutritious foods can greatly benefit a patient's food pattern.

Living conditions, too, may be very significant. This can be true whether a patient is living independently or in a nursing home. Nutrition is not a simple matter for individuals who are adjusting to the new atmosphere of an institution. Lack of appetite may reflect depression, discouragement, or withdrawal from the strange environment. Meals may be rejected if foods are very different from those to which the patient is accustomed or served without aesthetic considerations, and unhealthy attitudes toward food may develop. Unless a real effort is made to understand and to consider individual feelings, preferences, and cultural patterns, the patient's emotional reactions to his food may have serious consequences.

With other individuals there are other problems which frequently demand the attention of the physician if good nutrition is to be attained. Persons who live with their children often have to accommodate themselves to the family's food choices and may need help in arranging to have suitable food or meals. If a patient lives alone, there is always the question of whether he or she has the skill or the will to cook. Also, food patterns may be determined by facilities for refrigeration, cooking, storage, or marketing. The stores may be too remote, the transporting or the steps too exhausting. Planning and buying for just one or two is another task which often requires difficult adjustments and new learning. Even restaurants may not be a solution; sometimes they are too far away, especially in bad weather, too costly, or too lonely.

This hazard, loneliness, is among the most serious of all the challenges which face the elderly. As circumstances gradually reduce the circle of friends and family and the amount of available living space, the elderly patient is apt to grow more and more withdrawn, less and less interested in eating. Again the vicious circle enters the picture. Loss of appetite leads to poor food practices. Calories get out of balance, and essential nutrients are neglected, so the patient develops more anorexia and becomes progressively more malnourished and listless. Nutritional rehabilitation entails breaking this circle, with an attempt to find companionship for the patient to encourage him to eat and to help him enjoy mealtime.

The whole situation becomes more complicated when the doctor has to tackle not only poor food habits but also distorted attitudes. Understanding the psychological meaning of food, significant at every age, becomes of paramount importance in treatment of the elderly. By this period, rejection of food may indicate either a desire for self-destruction or a device to wrench attention from someone. On the other hand, others may find in food a last remaining pleasure, and so it assumes an undue importance.

The tendency of everyone to grow less flexible with age may also create problems. Patience and understanding are indispensable tools for the physician who hopes to break a patient's adherence to whims and prejudices. Such confidence in fads and fancies, overlaying the eternal hope of a quick return to youth and health, drives many an older person into the traps of quacks. Nutritional nonsense, fads, and fakes create a very serious economic and medical problem with the aging population. Unfortunately, older people with time to read and time to yearn spend disastrous sums from their meagre incomes on misleading books and bottles, pills, powders, and "health foods" filled with promises of rejuvenation and miraculous restoration to health.

One of today's greatest challenges to those concerned with nutritional rehabilitation is to counter misinformation with correct information. The physician needs to be aware of the lure and the cost of false or unnecessary dietary supplements and of his obligation to save the gullible aged from fads and fallacies.

The physician can be a countersalesman, teaching patients to distinguish between "health" foods which just exhaust the pocketbook and nutritious foods which bring health. This difference can be budget-saving and life-saving to patients in need of good nutrition and of optimum efficiency, comfort, and happiness "as life draws to a close."

A PATTERN FOR BALANCED MEALS

For some individuals it is enough to learn that good nutrition depends on sensible selection of the Basic Four foods. Others, however, may need specific suggestions about organizing meals, arranging menus, and making adaptions to fit special dietary and/or budgetary situations. These people can be greatly benefited if the physician can outline a simple plan such as the following sample pattern:

Breakfast
> Fruit or juice: This is a good time to supply vitamin C.
> Protein Food: Egg, cheese, or cereal with milk.
> Energy Food: Toast or roll.
> Spread: Butter or margarine or jam, according to need and preference.
> Beverage.

Main Meal (whether at noon or at night)
> Protein: Three to four ounces of meat, fish, or poultry.
> Energy Food: Potato or rice or macaroni or noodles or bread or a combination.

Vegetable: This can be cooked or raw or both.
Fruit or other dessert.
Beverage.

Lunch or Supper

Protein: Cheese or egg or slice of meat or poultry or small portion of fish.
Vegetable.
Energy Food: Similar to main-meal choice.
Spread: Butter or margarine, again according to need and preference.
Fruit.
Beverage.

This is a pattern which can be adjusted for each patient. Extras can be added and portion sizes increased or decreased according to individual need. This will also determine the amount and kind of bread and kind of spread which should be recommended, the amount and kinds of fats and oils, the type of dessert, the use of sugar and other sweets, and the type of beverage.

Choice and use of foods can be regulated by personal preference. They can be raw or cooked, combined in soups, stews, or casseroles—whatever is convenient and appealing. At the end of the day, though, the total intake should include all the items in the sample pattern and a sufficiency of dairy products.

The number of meals is flexible. If more than three seem desirable, the total allowance can be redistributed, permitting something between meals or at bedtime. The arrangement need not be rigid; what is of paramount importance is regularity. Older people who eat odd foods at odd hours and fill up on tea and toast or coffee and crackers inevitably show signs of poor nutrition.

Such careless practices or a patient's ignorance or his stubborn adherence to mistaken theories often hamper the doctor's efforts to improve a nutritional pattern. Success may rest on the physician's ability to build on the patient's good habits, to explain carefully the basis for suggested changes, and to give convincing reasons for relinquishing foolish notions. Among these are the prejudice against canned and frozen products, belief in the value of "fresh" foods or "red" meat, and the idea that foods must be bland and unappetizing because spices and flavorings are harmful.

Still another challenge is the elderly person who blames his poor nutrition on his limited income. In this instance the physician can make a significant contribution to his patient's nutritional rehabilitation simply by being aware that all too often both dollars and nutrients are lost through waste in buying, in cooking, and in use of leftovers. Knowing this, the doctor can sometimes be most helpful with just a few pointers which can at the same time bolster a patient's budget and also his nutrition.

For instance, as noted elsewhere, use of dry or evaporated milk can be a substantial money saver. Grade A in a can compared with grade C may give no more though it costs much more. Vitamin C is the same whether it comes from fresh, frozen, or canned products. In fact, with many foods, choice should be based on cost and not on type of processing. Also, many patients could save if they would learn to look at labels and to buy in less expensive, larger quantities, if the food could then be either eaten up or stored properly.

In purchasing protein, too, cost is no criterion of food value. Cheap meat may not be a bargain if it is chiefly bone and fat, but many thrifty specials make delicious dishes (especially with the aid of a grinder or tenderizer). Fish in season is often overlooked, and even the least costly liver is a rich source of protein, iron, and vitamins. Dried peas and beans or cereal and milk also stretch the food dollar and so does peanut butter, if the fat is no problem.

Proper selection of vegetables can also subtract costs and add food value in a day's intake. For instance, though lettuce is usually a luxury, just one serving of another leafy green vegetable such as spinach can provide a whole day's requirement of vitamin A. Potatoes, squash, and carrots are other vegetables which are high in nutritive content and relatively low in cost.

Value, then, is a matter of cost, content, and contribution to health. Wise choices depend upon skillful counsel. An informed and understanding physician, sensitive to all the complex factors involved, can guide his geriatric patient to the good food habits which are indispensable in dynamic maintenance therapy.

REFERENCES

1. STARE, F. J., and SHEA, J.: Nutritional needs of older people. *The Merck Report, 64,* 1955.
2. STARE, F. J.: Nutritional problems of advancing age. *Bull. N. Y. Acad. Med., 32:*284, 1956.
3. LYONS, J. S., and TRULSON, M. F.: Food practices of older people living at home. *J. Geront., 11:*66, 1956.
4. STARE, F. J.: Nutrition of the geriatric patient. *J. Amer. Geriat. Soc. 4:*744, 1956.
5. BLUMENTHAL, G. W.: Emotional aspects of feeding the aged. *J. Amer. Diet. Ass., 32:*829, 1956.
6. CHINN, A. B.: Some problems of nutrition in the aged. *JAMA, 162:*1511, 1956.
7. BEEUWKES, A. M.: Studying the food habits of the elderly. *J. Amer. Diet. Ass., 37:*215, 1960.
8. HASHIM, S. A.: The difficult patient—how do you feed him? *Nutr. Rev., 20:*1, 1962.
9. BASS, I.: Don't take fun out of food for the aged. *Mod. Hosp., 98:*140, 1962.
10. STARE, J. F.: Proper eating has become a science. *J. Amer. Geriat. Ass., 10:*737, 1962.
11. MAYER, J.: Nutrition in the aged. *Postgrad. Med., 32:*394, 1962.
12. TUNBRIDGE, R. E.: Right food for the right age. *J. Coll. Gen. Pract., 6:*49, 1963.
13. ROSS, C. H.: Nutrition in geriatrics. *J. Mich. Med. Soc., 62:*878, 1963.
14. And a happy old age. *Canad. Med. Ass. J., 89:*724, 1963.
15. WIGHTMAN, K. J. R.: Pitfalls in the management of the geriatric patient. *Appl. Ther., 6:*26, 1964.
16. OHLSON, M. A.: Food for the aging. *Med. Times, 92:*878, 1964.
17. *Recommended Dietary Allowances,* 6th revised ed., National Academy of Science, National Research Council, 1964.
18. WATKIN, D. M.: Food for the aging. *In Modern Nutrition in Health and Disease.* M. G. Wohl and R. S. Goodhart (Eds.), Philadelphia, Lea and F., 1963.
19. Food consumption and dietary levels of older households in Rochester, New York. *Home Economic Research Report,* No. 25, Agricultural Research Service, U. S. Department of Agriculture, 1965.
20. *A Guide to Nutrition and Food Service for Nursing Homes and*

Homes for the Aged. U. S. Department of Health, Education, and Welfare, June, 1965.

Pamphlets for the Elderly

1. KING, C. G., and BRITT, G.: *Food Hints for Mature People.* Nutrition Foundation, Inc., 1962.
2. *Your Age and Your Diet.* Chicago, AMA.

Chapter VII

PSYCHIATRIC ASPECTS OF MAINTENANCE[*] CARE OF THE AGED PATIENT

BERNARD A. STOTSKY

I N THE treatment of the geriatric patient, the individual needs and problems of the patient and the integration of the patient with his environment must be carefully weighed. The environment may consist of the patient's home, his family's residence, the hospital, nursing home, or home for the aged. The attitudes and reactions of other people to the patient in relation to the setting must also be considered. This is particularly important to the geriatric patient because, unlike other adults, the older patient is more dependent upon other people, such as members of the family or nurses, for protection and satisfaction of daily needs. As a result, the interrelationship of the patient with his social and physical environment is crucial in determining whether or not a patient can adjust successfully in a particular setting.

The pathogenic environment is characterized by little gaiety, laughter, or evidence of enjoyment of life. There is often swearing, shouting, or even worse, tomblike silence. Few people come and go. The smell of sweat and urine may be present.

Volunteers are eager to work with adolescents and young people or even with the physically handicapped if they are not too old, but it is hard to recruit volunteers to work with the aged. It is usually very difficult to find a parking place in front of a general hospital, sometimes in some communities in front of a mental hospital; this is rarely a problem in front

*The ideas in this paper were stimulated by research performed by the author under Grant MHO-1624-01 from the National Institute of Mental Health, U. S. Department of Health, Education, and Welfare.

of a nursing home or a home or hospital for the aged. Members of the family often find some "necessary business" which keeps them away from these settings. Yet there are many modern nursing homes with a cheerful, gay atmosphere; attractively furnished and clean rooms; and many ongoing activities.

Most younger adults lack rapport with aged people. It is hard to empathize with them. The problems they face are frightening—death, concern with increasingly deficient bodily functions, increasing financial dependency, and possibly loss of friends and relatives. One also sees an absence of concern (or, at best, superficial concern) by others for the patient. Children may visit because of feelings of guilt rather than genuine interest in the patient. The patient is aware of this and may react by becoming angry, sullen, withdrawn, or oversolicitious for the welfare of relatives who are really neglecting him. Care and responsibility for the patient is turned over to the state and the extended care facility. The patient sees this as rejection. He has to deal with what, in his eyes, is an impersonal agency whose representatives are insensitive to his needs. He may regard the agency as concerned with enforcing regulations and ignore the useful functions it serves by obtaining the full benefits to which the patient is entitled.

The overall result is that many patients settle down to a slow wait for death with progressive loss of mental functions. They become increasingly disoriented, confused, and focused around the immediate present. When their faculties are intact, they may become depressed and seclusive. At times they may become overly property-conscious in a desire to hang on to the few things which belong to them. Slowing of thought and activity leads to loss of purposive behavior. Patients who remain at home or with their families retire discretely to a point where they are least noxious to more vigorous members of the family. Naturally this situation deteriorates, and with the loss of significant functions the patient soon finds his physical presence rather difficult to bear. The suicide rate of patients over sixty is higher than the national average for other age groups. Retirement to homes for the aged and nursing homes where they will be with peers who face an equally bleak and equally hopeless future is often the only recourse. A process of labelling takes place. The more disturbed patients are diagnosed as psychotic and sent to mental hospitals where they, having been labelled as mental patients, are regarded as a breed apart.

The few who retain their faculties separate themselves as much as they can from these other patients and prefer to be considered as different. They are nevertheless keenly aware of their growing inadequacy and often stagnate mentally. One sees a lack of alertness or rather a redirection of interest and attention to one's body and to one's immediate needs. These patients can be endlessly boring to others by their recital of symptoms and feelings of malaise. This often infuriates the nursing staff in institutions who have to differentiate the crisis from the chronic situation. The patient "cries wolf" so often that when he truly has an acute symptom indicative of some change, the staff will not pay much attention to it and will regard it as just part of the patient's hypochondriacal concern. Some members of the nursing staff become hardened. Many become too depressed and leave the institutional settings for the aged. As a result, there is a great deal of turnover in these facilities. The attitude of staff is custodial and restrictive, but benevolent. Patients, when disturbed, are regarded as a threat even though (in most instances) they may be able to do very little physical damage. Soon the feeling develops that the outlook for these people is hopeless. The staff does not engage in much direct contact and activity with these patients. After all, why identify with someone who is going to die or leave you in the relatively near future?

In the past, the kind of nursing personnel who have worked in institutions for the aged has frequently been below the average for other facilities in skill and in rapport with patients. As indicated above, the personnel who are sensitive to the needs of these patients become depressed and often have to leave for their own mental health. Another factor which has to be considered is that most institutions for the aged have to run at a much lower cost than general hospitals and even the more modern and up-to-date mental hospitals. As a result, the drive for economy means that in many places a minimum number of staff is available for treating patients. The excess work load is itself quite discouraging, particularly to professional nursing personnel who have as their model a hospital situation in which staffing is more generous and skilled staff more available. Many professional personnel in nursing homes develop an inferiority complex and soon come to feel that they are not as good as the staff in other settings. They feel looked down upon. If they stay in nursing homes, they will often lose interest in their profession and become prey to other influences such as an inordinate desire to improve their financial position. In some cases the most competent nurses become administrators and give up their professional nursing duties, particularly in homes which can employ both an administrator and a nursing supervisor.

The desire to educate lower-echelon staff is lost by virtue of high turnover and in many instances by the caliber of personnel coming to work. The nursing home may serve as a place for drifters and people who have difficulty in keeping jobs. This is certainly not a healthy situation for the chronically ill patient who needs understanding, patience, and a high degree of skill in the area of interpersonal relationships. Fortunately, there has been a sharp upgrading of standards and of the caliber of nursing personnel in nursing homes so that more competent professional personnel are entering the field.

With elderly patients a vicious circle may occur: In reaction to feeling rejected, the patient becomes disturbed and alienated from others; the motivation to understand and treat the patient goes down. The patient may be turned over to institutional management. Many families will first try a nursing home or a home for the aged or admission to a general hospital. When the patient proves unmanageable in these places or if the symptoms are aggravated by the conditions which have been described above, he is transferred to a state mental hospital. The thought, of course, is that the patient needs the kind of discipline, control, and medical and nursing care which is available in state hospitals. As a matter of fact this is a fiction. The chronic wards of state hospitals are poorly staffed. The best and most highly skilled staff members are often concentrated in the reception units or the acute intensive treatment units. As a result, the patient is placed in an environment where he receives less care than elsewhere. For the patient who needs to be disengaged from a "hot" situation at home and needs less stimulation, this may be all right; however, many patients experience this as rejection. They feel abandoned and become depressed and even paranoid because they believe that they have been railroaded into an institution. This sudden shift from one setting to another may result in the patient's giving up or in hyperactivity or withdrawal into inactivity and unresponsiveness. The death rate in the first year following admission for aged patients in mental hospitals is high, ranging from 30 to 60 per cent for patients over sixty-five.

Medical care in mental hospitals is frequently less adequate than in general hospitals or the better nursing homes. If the patient survives, he has to adjust himself to an environment in which there is reduced stimulation and in which there or other patients who may be far more regressed than he. Once the family members believe that the patient is adequately taken care of, they are inclined to look at hospitalization as relief from a burden and may give up the idea of ever having the patient back home again. This results in the development of a pattern of chronic hospitalization and of withdrawal from contacts with others and with the activities of one's previous life. The patient will then adjust to the hospital, which becomes his home for life. At best, he may expect transfer to another kind of institution, a smaller one such as a nursing home, a rest home, or a home for the aged. This tends to introduce an element of chronicity into the patient's psychiatric picture. He develops the earmarks of the chronic patient and makes his adjustment to the institution rather than renewing older bonds with his family. Out of guilt the family may visit, but one notices that visits become less frequent the longer the patient stays in an institutional setting.

PSYCHOLOGICAL FACTORS

The whole process of disengagement involves separation from

one's previous pattern in many instances, departure from a familiar situation and entry into an alien setting. There are some people who make a virtue of this separation and stress the need for adjustment to a new life, with activities and relationships appropriate to this life. As a matter of fact, when one looks at the situation for most geriatric patients realistically, it is not a new life in any positive sense but rather a kind of twilight zone wherein the patient simply develops an institutional mode of adjustment or a pattern of waiting for death.

The issue of loss is a very great one. There is the loss of security, loss of status, loss of health, and most important, loss of significant people. Death of friends and relatives is a frequent occurrence. The patient must accept the inevitability of loss. This tends to produce a sense of helplessness and inadequacy, and a feeling of loss of control over the environment as well as increased sensitivity to disease and death. Intellectual deficits develop which are superimposed on the deficits characteristically associated with degenerative changes of old age, such as loss of memory functions, mild confusion, and disorientation. Ability to concentrate decreases, particularly in depressed patients. Patients may react with extreme apprehension, fear, and agitation. Somatic symptoms increase. The patient may manifest agitation, hyperactivity, noisiness, and boisterousness, which may make him vulnerable to exhaustion and to the aftereffects of exhaustion, such as cardiovascular failure or cerebrovascular accidents.

Anger and resentment develop which are difficult to express to others. The patient recognizes that he has no reasonable basis for these feelings. As a result the anger becomes directed inward. He becomes guilty for feeling angry and turns it against himself with self-reproaches, agitation, and in more extreme forms with delusions of self-accusation or ideas of imminent death. At a deeper level there is an unverbalized accusation against others for allowing him to get into this condition. In such situations, consultation and discussion are needed. In the more aggravated forms, hospitalization may be required.

BEHAVIOR MANIFESTATIONS OF
POOR ADJUSTMENT

The most common symptom of poor adjustment in the aged is depression in which the patient becomes slowed down in thought, speech, and activity as well as reporting depressed affect. He may develop vegatative symptoms such as loss of appetite, poor sleep patterns, and particularly early morning rising before 5 A.M. He loses interest in activity and in people and reports a general feeling of hopelessness and futility as well as a tendency to depreciate himself. One may also see withdrawn and sullen behavior. Patients become quite passive and dependent and adopt an attitude of helplessness and attachment to others which is characterized by demands on other people for care and attention. Sometimes these represent attempts to manipulate by focusing on one's own bodily needs. Depressed patients may endlessly elaborate these symptoms and consequently feel unable to undertake anything on their own responsibility.

Disturbed form of behavior may be a reaction of assaultiveness and aggressiveness, particularly on the part of people who are apprehensive and fearful of the intentions of others. In an extreme form one sees this in paranoid, suspicious behavior in which patients become assaultive and aggressive toward specific people whom they regard as wanting to harm them. Sometimes the assaultive behavior will be periodic and occur during periods of confusion. The evening is always a difficult time for the elderly patient. At night when there is less light, confusion becomes intensified. Aggressive and boisterous behaviors increase toward persons as does destructive behavior toward property. Patients, partly out of confusion and partly out of a desire to leave an unpleasant situation, will wander off or may attempt to escape. They often wander into other rooms or try to get into bed with other people. In view of the rather constricted living space of most patients, this kind of intrusion is taken with ill grace by the person whose property has been invaded, and altercations may ensue.

Some patients may increase their alcoholic consumption or be less able to manage the same amount of alcohol. Others will attempt to obtain drugs. Quite often these people have a history of drug ingestion and are habituated to such drugs. Under careful surveillance, these patients may not be able to procure quantities of drugs which they want and may become irritable and difficult to manage until given the medication or some substitute. This is also true of alcoholics. As a result they do poorly in nursing homes where stricter supervision is exercised than at home. Patients may become boisterous and act child- ishly and silly. Some react to authority by becoming infantile or by behaving in a way counter to their own prior morals and values. Sometimes sexual behavior has a resurgence during this period. Patients who are far past the age of ability will attempt to become involved in sexual activities (either of a homosexual or heterosexual character) with other patients.

There is an increase in symptoms of physical illness. Patients lose weight, in large part attributable to decreased or sporadic food intake. There is a loss of appetite and also a loss of interest in eating and in the performance of daily activities. Hygiene and personal grooming suffer. Disturbance of sleep and some- times even a reversal of sleep pattern occur. Slowing of peris- talsis in old age may give rise to constipation or to increased difficulty in digesting food. Respiratory difficulties due to changes in pulmonary tissue are often seen and may aggravate psychiatric symptoms which are present. Thus, a patient who has been asthmatic in his adult years and becomes emphy- sematous may become agitated during these periods because he fears, with some justification, that he may die or that he may not be properly handled.

The physically ill patient, especially the patient suffering from cardiovascular and respiratory diseases, shows increased concern about physical condition. Such a patient may be reluctant to take walks or to engage in any strenuous physical activity. Some patients become so fearful of possible physical consequences that they give up taking care of themselves, particularly in the areas of dress and bathing. Ambulatory patients are sometimes hardest hit; many will either take to bed or take to sitting for long periods of time because of fear of complications.

In the aging, this intermixture of physical and mental symptoms results in an accentuation of both. The patient becomes more vulnerable to infection and to illnesses than the younger person who is stronger, better able to take care of himself, and leads a less sedentary life. The presence of other aged people, particularly in an institutional setting, always tends to keep in the forefront physical as well as mental illness. The patient has a higher expectation of becoming ill and is more sensitive to early symptoms of illness.

It is highly important to differentiate between patients who suffer from organic disease of the brain and patients who have a functional disorder. The major differentiating factors to consider are listed in textbooks but will be briefly reviewed here. These relate primarily to intellectual deficits such as the presence of confusion, disorientation, loss of recent memory, loss of ability to concentrate, loss of judgment, loss of insight, and loss of abilities in specific areas such as in handling numerical operations or in reasoning. Patients with these deficits are usually on a progressive, irreversible course. Nevertheless, they often have a functional overlay with symptoms of depression, agitation, and paranoid delusion. These latter can be treated and alleviated. Patients may be particularly subject to marked fluctuations of mood. Their mental status may appear worse with these emotional upsets than the brain syndrome itself would suggest. With appropriate treatment, marked improvement may be noted.

The functional disorders are mainly related to disorders of affect such as depression, involutional reactions, or mixed reactions which involve both paranoid and depressive symptoms. One occasionally sees personality disorders and even a schizophrenia of late onset, although the latter is relatively rare over sixty-five. There is an abundance of psychosomatic disorders. Here one must differentiate between people who have a physical disease and who may be exaggerating it slightly from those who have no known organic disease and whose symptoms reflect a kind of psychological defense mechanism for dealing with a problem in the environment. The latter requires careful evaluation and the possible removal of the cause. On the other hand, this preoccupation with one's own bodily function may be an excellent defensive gesture to protect the patient from a feeling of hopelessness, uncontrolled fear, or abandonment. In this sense, somatic symptoms serve as an adaptive mechanism. By concentrating his attention on his bodily state, the patient protects himself from a more pathogenic psychological reaction. At times this defense needs to be supported. At other times it needs to be gradually removed and replaced with more constructive modes of adjusting, such as recreational and rehabilitative activities.

PSYCHIATRIC EVALUATION

Psychiatric evaluation really has to be tailored to the particular situation. For example, if a psychiatrist or a family physician is called in a state of crisis to deal with a problem which has arisen recently or is the result of some acute situation, it is important both to treat the patient and to obtain a good history of the environmental events which have occurred, particularly events related to loss of important people and sudden changes in the patient's life. The latter would include physical illness and changes in physical functioning. The kinds of crises which demand psychiatric attention are acute depressions, manic episodes, the sudden onset of paranoid behavior, delirium, confusion, suicidal attempts, or attacks on others. The physician must intervene quickly and act decisively in these situations and at the same time keep an eye open to the precipitating causes.

It takes courage to keep an acutely disturbed patient in his environment; many untapped resources can often be utilized. For example, a depressed and at times even a suicidal patient may conceivably be treated at home if the family is interested enough to exert additional effort in behalf of the patient. Just the intention and willingness of the family to help is often interpreted as a favorable sign by the patient. Many patients respond when the family mobilizes itself to deal with the crisis. Hospitalization serves to protect the patient and quite often the physician and family as well. However, it may not always be in the best interests of the patient. If the family, with the support of a physician, can reconstitute itself to deal with the situation, hospitalization may be either delayed, avoided, or certainly shortened in duration by appropriate management of the crisis. This may require medication and also special care.

It would actually be most useful if hospitals had units for the temporary care of patients either on a daytime and nighttime basis or for twenty-four hours without the highly involved admission and processing procedures which exist now. As the patient pulls himself together and the family focuses its attention on the patient's problems, ways to deal with them can be found which may be lost if responsibility for management of the patient is turned over entirely to the hospital and the hospital's physician, who may not know the patient. This is a very important factor to consider. The psychiatrist must be mindful not only of what he and the family physician can do but also of what other community resources are available. For example, visiting nurses and public health nurses can be of great assistance in dealing with these problems. Social caseworkers, particularly in such agencies as family and children's services and other community agencies, may be of great help to the family and to the patient himself.

Another type of psychiatric evaluation is a routine assessment of progressive deficit usually in memory and in intellectual functions, with subsequent confusion and disorientation. The family may have tolerated this change for as long as it could. When it no longer feels able to do so, the physician is called in. This type of consultation involves an evaluation of the mental status of the patient to determine whether a chronic brain syndrome is present or whether a more acute condition exists. In such a case, if the patient has not been followed carefully by his own physician, it is necessary to make a thorough physical examination in order to rule out the presence of physical disease. There are many undiagnosed physical diseases which may contribute both to acute and chronic brain syndromes; for example, respiratory disease, malnutrition, and acute infectious diseases in almost any system of the body.

Another possibility which must be considered is the presence of a neoplasm. If a patient has not been seen on a regular basis by his family physician, it is usually advisable to hospitalize the patient in order that diseases of a neurological character may be ruled out as soon as possible. Involved may be a detailed work-up including x-ray of the skull, lumbar puncture, electroencephalograms, and if necessary, pneumoencephalograms, ventriculograms, or arteriograms. Radiological studies of other systems of the body may also be necessary as well as the usual medical work-up involving evaluation of various systems of the body, both through physical examination and laboratory evaluation. Brain scans, using radioisotopes, are helpful.

Much can also be said for prophylactic psychiatric evaluation before the onset of serious mental illness. The psychiatrist in performing a mental status exam can obtain reliable data in many cases. He can be helped by a thorough neurological examination as well as by a psychological work-up. Psychological tests have a high degree of precision alone or in combination with the EEG in detecting the presence of organic brain disease.

In many instances without such evaluations one does not have a good picture, except through the distorted accounts from the family and the patient, of the premorbid state of the patient. Is the change gradual? Is the patient much different from what he was ten, fifteen, or twenty years ago, or even two years ago? These questions are answered only in a speculative way when a psychiatrist is called upon *either in* a crisis or as a result of a chronic behavioral change which has just been noted by the family. As a matter of fact, when the patient finally reaches the hospital and is evaluated there, other factors have intervened such as the transfer of the patient from home to hospital. The evaluation performed at that time may reflect his reaction to transfer from home or from some extended-care facility to a mental hospital. As a result the psychiatrist may have to assess the impact of hospitalization on the patient as well as the patient's condition itself. For this reason it is probably well for the patient to have a mental health examination in addition to a physical checkup on a routine basis. Yearly examinations may be too frequent, but it would certainly seem advisable for the patient to undergo an evaluation of mental status and psychological testing as well as laboratory studies every five years, or more often as indicated.

To be considered also is the effect of segregation on the patient when he is removed from the community and put in a setting where there are other people who are more or less disturbed than he. The patient is subject to a kind of social contagion: Symptoms spread and disturbed behavior spreads. Patients tend to imitate others in their environment. They also tend to be treated in a special way by others. Thus, if a patient is treated with the expectation that he will become disturbed, he may comply more readily than if the expectation is that he will take care of himself and act in a more normal way. All this must be considered from the standpoint of both evaluation and disposition.

TREATMENT

There are really three aspects to treatment which must be considered: The first is psychological treatment which in its broadest sense involves both psychotherapy of various kinds and psychologically oriented activities. The second category is somatic therapy wherein pharmacological agents or other special agents such as electroshock are introduced to help the patient. A third category of treatment is via the milieu—manipulation of the environment to help the patient. In any treatment situation, the three are usually interrelated and integrated. Simply for purpose of exposition they will be considered separately, though obviously the wise physician makes use of all three modalities.

Psychological Treatment

The broad aims of psychological treatment are to assist the patient in regaining interest in activity and in solving problems for himself. The patient's primary problems are boredom, loneliness, and a sense of loss. Patients do not know what to do with themselves. They feel alone, deserted, abandoned, and often do not have the energy or the initiative to undertake activities. Sometimes they will not relate to other patients in an institution and will refuse to associate with them. There is much which can be done at the subprofessional level. Group activities and recreational activities can be encouraged. Games such as bingo, cards, or activities involving groups—hootenannies, small work projects, and so on—can help a great deal. Contact with a volunteer on a regular basis can do much to combat loneliness. Volunteer-organized group work involving patients doing things with each other, even if it is only walking to the store or buying something to eat in a restaurant, and doing things for other people can be therapeutic. A volunteer can go a long way toward removing the feeling of loneliness.

Families can be helpful, but they can also be a major hindrance. Quite often, relationships with the family have become very disturbed, and the family members may need some guidance in approaching the patient and in dealing with both the patient's feelings and their own feelings. Members of the family can be very useful in visiting, in doing things with the patient, and in talking about things which are of interest to the patient. They can also aggravate conflicts which exist and increase tension in the nursing home by their demands and their eccentric behavior.

A very important factor in the lives of aged patients is economic insecurity. One aspect of psychological treatment is to do something to remove this feeling of insecurity by lessening economic burdens and by helping the patient to utilize resources which are available for this purpose. Motility and competence are extremely important in the aged group. Ways can be devised to foster motility by making it necessary and at the same time possible for the patient to get around so that he has to do things for himself through movement and through activity. One can provide situations which help give the patient a sense of competence. For example, if a patient can operate a motion picture projector, he can show films to the other members of the group. He may help in chores around the home such as making his own bed, preparing snacks, and cleaning up his own area. Quite often, nurses and family members overprotect and infantilize the patient by not allowing him to do anything. On the other hand, one must avoid the other extreme in which the patient is exploited while family members or staff members sit around and use the patient to enable them to avoid work.

An important ingredient of psychological treatment is the

aggressive practice of preventive medicine in the sense of helping the patient to avoid disease by appropriate care and by self-care measures which give the patient an increased sense of competence and a feeling of reduced vulnerability. Little things can be done to increase the patient's orientation such as having a calendar to remind him of the date and discussing current events with him to keep him up-to-date and to reinforce the memory of recent events.

From a therapeutic standpoint the concentration on television in many nursing homes and extended-care facilities is useless and sometimes detrimental to patient welfare. Staff and patients take the easy way out in this respect. Patients are allowed to sit in front of the television for hours at a time. If one watches closely, he may see that the patient is not really concentrating on the television program but simply sitting and staring at the set. He may not even bother to look but simply sits there because he has nothing better to do. The staff may feel that the patient is actually doing something, but in reality he is not. It would probably be much better to foster group discussions and games, even when at times this may seem stilted and artificial, to keep the patient alert, participating, and active. Another measure which can be of great help psychologically is to provide adequate lighting and company at night. Volunteers come for the most part during the daytime when the patient has relatively less need for company, whereas at night a real person is needed to replace the imaginary people who often exist in the minds of patients at night. Adequate lighting helps to counteract confusion and disorientation.

Finally, from a psychological standpoint, it is important to have healthy and stable family members at home and healthy and stable staff members in institutions. Hospitals and nursing homes with high turnover are subject to many instances of emotionally disturbed behavior, accidents to both patients and staff, and probably an increased incidence of physical illness. Psychologists, psychiatrists, and caseworkers consulting to nursing homes and nurses working within nursing homes should pay a great deal of attention to the needs of staff and should discuss problems with staff. Many nursing homes lack basic information for dealing with patients. While not all staff members are reliable, there are many who are motivated to work better with patients if they know more about them and have help in dealing with their problems. Sometimes one has to be didactic and have regularly scheduled weekly or biweekly conferences to discuss problems of management both for specific patients and for patients in general. Unstructured sessions without agenda may not go over well because of the low level of information and weak organizational structure. Some personnel react to vagueness and ambiguity by becoming upset or rejecting such situations. The staff's needs for concrete information and for techniques to deal with crises in nursing homes and in homes for the aged are very great. In working with staff, one must take particular notice of the need for understanding and of the need for help with immediate problems.

Psychotherapy

Long-term intensive psychotherapy is probably not very useful for most aged patients. There are some who can benefit from an exploration of basic motivations with a view to enlarging their understanding of themselves. However, most patients probably need a form of psychotherapy oriented around particular personal issues and problems; for example, in adjusting to a new setting in a nursing home or hospital or in dealing with a newly developed physical or mental disability. They have a need for mastery and for support from strong figures in dealing with problems arising in relation to other patients and staff members.

In the office, brief ten- to thirty-minute therapy sessions are most useful. Patients become restless and often run out of material if a longer period is required. A great deal of attention must be paid to the intellectual status of the patient. Patients who are completely intact intellectually and still respond with a great deal of affect toward issues in their lives can often spend more time than thirty minutes and may even benefit from hour-long contacts with the psychiatrically trained physician or other mental health professionals.

The transference situation is such that it does not lend itself easily to interpretation. The therapist often uses aspects of the patient's reaction to him, whether in an attempt to control the therapy or in an attempt to develop a kind of childlike dependence on the therapist, to help the patient with a current problem rather than to increase his understanding of himself. The issues brought up in treatment are many but are particularly oriented to loss, separation, and coming to terms with the problem of death as well as personal insecurities, economic insecurities, or unsatisfied needs. The problem of understanding and being understood is very important, particularly when the patient is in a setting where people are too busy to spend much time with him.

A broader consideration in psychotherapy is that of supervision of staff people who come in contact with the patient and that of dealing with the family of the patient. In treatment of the aged, intensive work can be done with other family members in group sessions or in individual sessions. Again one must consider in an institutional setting both the family and the surrogate family such as staff members and nursing personnel.

Group psychotherapy has been valuable in the experience of Wolff (1), Linden (2), and more recently Honigfeld *et al.* (3). Group sessions oriented around problems of motivation and the discussion of problems which patients may share in common, particularly day-to-day problems, can be very helpful. Besides the skills which group psychotherapy ordinarily involves, the therapist requires patience and tolerance of slow movement and of eccentricity in patients. Very often, patients need to be reminded that a session is being held and encouraged each time to come. There may be a failure of recall from one session to the next and relatively little carry-over of themes from the previous hour. The same material is touched on again and again, much more often than in group therapy with younger people.

Conjoint family therapy may be helpful particularly when there are some tensions between the patient and his family. These have to be handled carefully because family skeletons, which have been kept in the closet and are released in such situations, can produce extreme disturbance both for the patient and for his family. In some instances it is necessary to let in a little bit of fresh air and deal with some of these issues; however, this is a delicate business. Sometimes the patient needs to be spared the tensions arising in sessions with the family. A tremendous amount of emotion can be expressed. Participants may be disturbed for a long period afterwards. A great deal of constructive work can nevertheless be accomplished. When one considers the theme of the family's feelings of guilt for placing the patient in an institution and the patient's unexpressed anger toward the family, a clearing of the air may result. Such a technique can be useful but involves the highest order of skill in management and in terms of the timing of such sessions. Flexibility in combining individual and family therapy sessions is a highly desirable way of proceeding.

Finally, one must consider spiritual needs. Clergymen can be extremely useful to older patients. A reawakening of religious feeling in the aged often occurs at the same time as an avoidance of the aged by the clergy for reasons which are not entirely clear. Clergy have often been reluctant to work with aged persons, disconcerting to those coming from a religious background and needing the support and sustenance which the clergy can give. Regular religious services and the giving of the sacraments, when the patient's faith demands it, can be very therapeutic.

Some homes are quite successful in creating a religious atmosphere, so that patients are constantly preoccupied with assisting themselves and others to prepare for death in an appropriate manner. While this can be depressing to some patients, it aids others to flourish in a setting where the performance of religious duties and observances is accepted as part of the social environment. Moreover, many patients, particularly those who were born and educated around the turn of the century, may distrust psychiatrists and other mental health professionals and may be able to communicate more easily with a clergyman. The background of the patient as well as the patient's mental status is highly important here and must be considered. Surprisingly enough, many otherwise deteriorated patients respond appropriately in the area of religious observance. In this sense it can be used as psychological therapy to increase activity and to foster the development of adequate daily routine. It also helps to counteract the boredom and the loneliness which one sees in the aged, particularly the institutionalized aged.

Somatic Therapy

The pharmacological treatment of aged patients is extremely widespread and is often abused. That is not to say that the majority of such patients are not being appropriately medicated. Titration of dosage of medication for the aged requires care. One encounters idiosyncratic reactions or side reactions to drugs. Probably older patients are more vulnerable to toxic reactions. Once the acute phase of the illness is passed, less than optimal attention is paid to the pharmacological treatment of elderly patients. Patients may be put on a maintenance dose of drugs and then suddenly become sensitive to them. They may also gradually become more sensitive and develop side effects which are not attended to until the patient is fairly far along toward toxicity. There are also special considerations such as the relative intolerance of aged patients to many agents. Some patients react paradoxically to barbiturates and other sedative drugs with excitement and confusion and in a few instances with convulsions. Sensitivity to phenothiazine drugs may be manifested by extrapyramidal effects such as dystonia, akathisia, dyskinesia, and in extreme cases opisthotonos and oculogyric crisis. These are often difficult to manage.

A great hazard in the use of tranquilizing drugs is hypotension. Many patients will have a syncopal episode following a dose of chlorpromazine or thioridazine. They may be treated for stroke or may actually develop stroke following ingestion of a large dose of such drugs. Seizures and excitement will occasionally occur in response to tranquilizing medication. Blood dyscrasias such as leukopenia, more rarely agranulocytosis or aplastic anemia may develop. Patients may also develop liver complications with jaundice. Serum alkaline phosphatase levels and enzyme levels (SGOT, LDH) may be elevated. Patients may overreact to relatively small doses and become underactive and somnolent. Since they are not disturbing to the staff in this condition, they may not draw much attention until the patient gradually lose weight, lose appetite, and seem to drift off into semicomatose states.

Such reactions as nasal congestion, dry mouth, miosis or mydriasis, constipation, difficulty in urinating, perspiration, and headache are common. Dermatologic reactions commonly include mild urticarial-type rashes and photosensitivity. Sometimes an exfoliative dermatitis may occur. Patients in long-term therapy may show pigmentation changes on the skin ranging from slight darkening to a slate gray. Deposition of pigment may occur on the cornea and lens, resulting in opacities on the latter. The question of visual changes is still unresolved. The drugs are contraindicated in severely depressed or comatose states.

It is not unusual to find patients being overmedicated. Some patients in institutional settings may have as many as ten to fifteen drugs, all taken the same day. Quite often these patients may be on the edge of toxicity or may have developed symptoms reflecting drug overdosage. Drugs will potentiate the effect of other drugs: for example, phenothiazines potentiate barbiturates, alcohol, antihistamines, and narcotics. In such instances one may see iatrogenic confusion, dulling, and oversedation as well as the onset of other symptoms and signs such as low blood pressure, increased pulse rate, and respiratory depression. Over a long period of time, addiction or habituation to drugs may result so that patients require large dosages and may show withdrawal effects when taken off the drugs. When one encounters a patient suffering from "polypharmacy," the use of many drugs concurrently for ill-defined symptoms, it is advisable to take the patient off all drugs gradually and observe the effects. One of the results of this procedure may be an improvement in the patient's psychiatric condition.

A question with patients who are emotionally disturbed, confused, and disoriented is whether to use drugs at all. Some drugs thought to be relatively safe, such as chlordiazepoxide and meprobamate, may occasionally aggravate confusion and disorientation rather than sedate. This is something which can be quite disturbing to the patient and result in serious consequences such as falls and fractures. In addition, one must also consider the fact that aged patients are sensitive to drug effects, so small doses can often be very effective. Thus trifluoperazine may be given in doses of one and two milligrams rather than in five or ten milligrams with salutary effects. It is advisable also not to give too much at one time unless a patient is extremely agitated and disturbed. Smaller doses can often result in alleviation of the condition. If a drug is being given for the first time or has an uncertain effect, it is advisable to obtain vital signs before administration of the drug and one and two hours after administration. If a patient has to be given intramuscular or even intravenous medication, it is advisable to observe the patient carefully. Syncopal episodes may occur or there may be more chronic effects of drugs.

Specific Drugs

The most commonly used medications in psychiatry are the tranquilizers. Essentially there are two kinds of tranquilizers. The minor tranquilizers such as chlordiazepoxide, diazepam, meprobamate, and related drugs are useful for patients who are intact intellectually and not psychotic but who experience anxiety and its somatic concomitants, particularly difficulty in sleeping. In many instances among elderly patients they may tend to increase confusion. They are of little value in dealing with psychotic manifestations. Patients may become incontinent, disoriented, and more disturbed. Quite often a bedtime dose of meprobamate, 400 mg, repeated once during the night if necessary, may help induce a restful night's sleep without recourse to barbiturates or hypnotic drugs. Recent studies show that meprobamate is habit-forming and that, with continued use, tolerance develops. For more disturbed behavior, particularly for psychotic manifestations such as paranoid thinking, delusions, hallucinations, hyperactivity, and aggressive behavior, it is advisable to use the phenothiazine drugs.

Usually 50 to 100 mg dosages of chlorpromazine two to four times a day, given at four-hour intervals, are enough to handle most disturbed behavior. If necessary one can go higher to 600 to 800 mg per day with caution. The advantage of chlorpromazine is its wide dose range, from 25 mg to 2,000 mg. The side effects are the ones described above for phenothiazine drugs. Of major concern in the aged are the hypotensive and Parkinson-like effects. The latter are easily controlled by anti-Parkinson agents: trihexyphenidyl, benztropine mesylate, biperiden, and procyclidine. The former are controlled by lowering dosage or by switching to piperazine series drugs such as trifluoperazine, perphenazine, and fluphenazine. Thioridazine, a piperidine drug, has been found useful, and it has almost the same effect in about the same dosage as chlorpromazine. The safe maximum dosage of thioridazine is 800 mg per day. Usually it is given in 25 to 50 mg doses, distributed over four-hour periods. It comes in a concentrate but not in injectable form. The side effects of thioridazine are similar to those of chlorpromazine. Pigmentary retinopathy has been observed among patients taking 1,600 mg or more per day over an extended period. For this reason, dosage of more than 800 mg per day is felt to be inadvisable. Thioridazine has a marked hypotensive effect and may be a little more risky in patients with cardiovascular disease or in patients who are more vulnerable to syncopal episodes. Therefore, blood pressure readings before and one and two hours after administration of thioridazine and chlorpromazine are recommended.

Chlorprothixene is a modified phenothiazine with a thioxanthene nucleus (double bond substituted for nitrogen atom) which is supposed to be effective for agitation. It is useful but tends to have less effect on acutely disturbed behavior of psychotic patients than chlorpromazine and thioridazine. It is available in a form which can be given intramuscularly. The side effects of chlorprothixene are very similar to those observed above for other phenothiazine drugs except that long-range pigmentary and ocular changes have not been reported. The piperazine forms of the phenothiazines are useful for the same kinds of behavior but have less immediate sedative action and may, therefore, be less effective in dealing with episodes of agitation. However, when one has to deal with chronic paranoid behavior or with apathy and preoccupation with hallucinations and delusions, these drugs are effective and reasonably safe. The most commonly used drugs are trifluoperazine, which comes in 1-, 2-, 5-, and 10-mg sizes; perphenazine, which comes in 2-, 4-, 8-, and 16-mg sizes; and fluphenazine, which comes in .25-, 1-, 2.50-, 5-, and 10-mg doses. These drugs have less of a sedating effect; therefore, the patient may appear to be more alert. However, they produce more severe extrapyramidal effects and usually have to be given along with anti-Parkinson agents. One milligram of the latter twice a day or two milligrams twice a day are usually sufficient to combat the side effects. However, if these effects are severe and are not sufficiently controlled, clearly the treatment of choice is to reduce the dose of the drug in question or to change to a different phenothiazine. Thioridazine and chlorprothixene are thought to produce fewer side effects.

Other phenothiazine drugs such as carphenazine and promazine are useful but tend to have less therapeutic effect in equivalent dosages than the drugs mentioned above. Promazine is used most commonly in general practice and may be effective for most symptoms. In cases of severe agitation, particularly for paranoid patients, it is probably advisable to use chlorpromazine or thioridazine. Prochlorperazine, a piperazine derivative, is used for tranquilization and also as an antiemetic. The drug has essentially the same effects as the others but also tends to produce a large number of side effects in large dosages. Patients on phenothiazines usually have an increased appetite. Excess weight gain may occur from this or from fluid retention. An adequate, balanced diet as well as vitamins, particularly for alcoholics or others whose disorders are complicated by alcoholism, is desirable.

For depression which is not characterized by extreme agitation or by suicidal behavior, there are a large number of antidepressant drugs available. The monoamine oxidase inhibitors such as phenelzine, nialamide, isocarboxazid, and tranylcypromine tend to be used less now because of the increased incidence of side effects such as hypotension, blood dyscrasias, hepatic dysfunction, and potentiation of other drugs. The more widely used agents are drugs which are related to the phenothiazines. These are imipramine, amitriptyline, nortriptyline, and desipramine. The dosages vary. Imipramine and amitriptyline come in 10- and 25-mg sizes and in an injectable solution.

Dose range is from 10 to 200 mg per day with a fair degree of safety, provided that the patient is not sensitive to the drug. There is some controversy as to which of the drugs is more effective regardless of dosage. More experience has accumulated with imipramine and amitriptyline. These drugs should not be used in conjunction with MAO inhibitors. At least several days should elapse before these drugs are used to replace MAO inhibitors and vice versa.

The side effects are fine tremor, hypotension or paradoxical hypertension, headache, jitteriness, excitement, nausea, dizziness, anorexia, dry mouth, nasal congestion, perspiration, skin rash, tachycardia, blurring of vision, constipation, numbness, and tingling. Rarely, seizures may occur. High doses may cause confusion and activate paranoid, delusional states of maniclike excitement. Amitriptyline may cause drowsiness. Extrapyramidal effects occur and are treated in the same way as with phenothiazines. Blood dyscrasias and hepatic dysfunction are rare. There is the danger with these drugs, just as there is with phenothiazines, of more severe complications such as myocardial infarctions and cerebral accidents. This risk must be weighed against the psychiatric picture and the needs of the patient. Where there is a question, a complete physical work-up should be done, with particular attention to the patient's cardiovascular status.

In cases of agitation or of manic excitement, it is advisable to use phenothiazines. Antidepressants are contraindicated. Chlorpromazine seems to be the most popular drug in treating manic states. New drugs which are being used are haloperidol and triperidol. These seem to have the same range of therapeutic effects and side effects as the phenothiazines. For manic-depressive reactions, lithium has been reported effective in some cases.

For patients with refractory depressions, particularly for those who are psychotically depressed and for whom there is a major risk of suicide or death from debilitation or malnutrition, and also for patients who are stuporous, whether due to depression or to catatonic withdrawal, electroshock therapy is the treatment of choice. The patient should not be kept waiting too long before the introduction of such therapy. It has a definite place in the treatment of such patients and may be life-saving. Usually the effects of such therapy will be manifested after several shock treatments. It is rare for some beneficial effects not to be manifested after ten treatments. A reasonable series of treatments would be ten, although in some cases it may be advisable to have periodic shock treatments, for example, on a monthly basis.

In addition, ECT can be combined with pharmacological therapy so that the patient may be taken out of a deep depression with shock treatment but may be maintained on antidepressant drugs or in some instances on phenothiazines where agitation and hyperactivity are in the forefront. One factor to consider is that phenothiazines may tend to deepen a depression. If a patient goes from agitation to a very deep depression which does not seem to yield to treatment, consideration should be given to taking the patient off drugs, particularly if he is on phenothiazines. This step obviously involves a thorough evaluation from a clinical standpoint.

Another mode of approach to the use of the pharmacological agents is combined treatment. The use of phenothiazines with antidepressant drugs has become quite common, and some drugs such as Triavil® (perphenazine and amitriptyline) are being marketed in a convenient form. However, physicians may prefer to make their own selection of dosages of antidepressants and phenothiazines, and these may not necessarily be the drug company's. In addition, the dosage of each drug may have to be controlled individually. However, where a combination is appropriate, it means that fewer pills have to be taken, and probably less resistance will be encountered from the patient. Cases of depression in which severe anxiety is present may be beneficially treated by these means.

However, one must keep in mind that the side effects and complications may be increased when two related drugs such as imipramine and chlorpromazine are being used. The patient's vulnerability to accident, to toxicity, or to increased side effects is increased by combining drugs. Insofar as possible, it is essential to avoid the combination of phenothiazines with barbiturates. The phenothiazines potentiate the barbiturate effect and may lead to very undesirable consequences such as comatose states or even cerebrovascular accidents.

The danger also exists that one may attempt to treat symptoms purely with drugs rather than investigate the psychological basis for such symptoms. The psychiatrist should thoroughly explore the patient's history, particularly with respect to recent events, to determine what can be done by other than pharmacological means.

As indicated above, ECT can be very valuable, particularly in cases of severe depression and even in some depressed individuals with paranoid coloring. This treatment should be carefully administered with the use of anesthesia and muscle relaxants. A currently popular form involves the use of methohexital or in some cases thiopental with succinylcholine. It is advisable to administer ECT in the hospital or in a clinical setting where an anesthesiologist as well as a psychiatrist is available, particularly among the aged where the possibility of accident and complications is greater than for younger patients. Electroshock therapy has been administered successfully to patients up to ninety years of age; in the author's experience, one patient with second-degree heart block was able to undergo a series of shock treatments with very careful monitoring of respiration and level of anesthesia.

One of the chronic complaints among the aged is insomnia. The problem of relief with medication is a challenge. Barbiturates can be used as well as paraldehyde and chloral hydrate, Chloral hydrate tends to be less effective but is relatively safe and seems to have some effect among patients with mild sleep disorders. Paraldehyde presents many problems particularly because of its relationship to alcohol. Barbiturates often produce paradoxical effects and may be hazardous especially when people get up in a confused state during the night, increasing the tendency to fall. One does not escape this problem with other drugs but must rely on clinical experience. Meprobamate, 400 mg at bedtime and possibly repeated once during the night, frequently is effective. It also comes in a 200-mg size which may be adequate for the needs of many aged people.

There are drugs such as glutethimide which act in much the

same way as barbiturates do. Although somewhat weaker in their action than the barbiturates, ethchlorvynol, methyprylon, and ethinamate are effective in treating mild insomnia. It is a little harder for an aged patient to become overdosed with these drugs though it does occur and can be life-threatening. One does not escape the problems of addiction with these drugs. The dosage must be adapted to the response of the aged person to such drugs. The standard weight formula is not completely adequate; one must individualize the prescription and be prepared for idiosyncratic responses. Formulas have been advanced using weight and body surface, but, for the present at least, a useful way to proceed is to titrate the drug dosage in relation to the effects it produces on the patient.

Since many aged patients require tranquilization during the day, an adequate distribution of dosage such that the patient gets a late evening dose of a drug like chlorpromazine or meprobamate may be adequate to insure a restful sleep. One can actually give a bedtime dose of such drugs which will facilitate sleep. Introduction of an additional drug is avoided and this enables the staff of an institution or the family members to establish a simple routine for administering medication.

In administering psychoactive drugs, one must be careful to note what other drugs the patient is taking. Practically any drug the patient takes, regardless for what condition, will produce central nervous system effects. Thus digitalis, quinidine, diuretics, and other commonly used drugs including pain relievers produce central nervous system effects. There is the danger of a synergistic effect of these drugs on the psychoactive drugs. Thus, drowsiness, fatigue, confusion, central nervous system depression, and in some cases hyperactivity and hallucinations may result. Therefore, if one is confronted with drug toxicity in a patient, it is necessary to evaluate the patient's total medicational regime as well as his condition to determine whether or not some drug or combination of drugs is the culprit.

Many patients, particularly in homes for the aged and in nursing homes where the physician either comes on call or sees the patient at long intervals and where prescriptions are more or less automatically renewed, are on a wide variety of drugs which are continued long beyond the need simply because no one discontinues the order. A dangerous situation can thus result, particularly in someone who does not have much physical reserve and may be vulnerable to infection or to upset of vital functions.

The Institutionalization of the Aged

The milieu or the environment around many aged people is conducive to a kind of chronicity and regression. Patients become apathetic. They remain isolated. They tend to deteriorate because of the institutionally imposed passivity, dependence, and separation from people outside the institution. Therefore, it is important for staff in an institutional setting to set as a goal the creation of an atmosphere which counteracts these trends. It is important to introduce or to reintroduce normal activities on a gradual basis. One can start with self-care and self-grooming, then introduce chores so that the patient is doing things for himself without necessarily becoming involved in them as a vocation. Trips to supermarkets, to movies, shopping trips, parties, picnics, games and visits on a regular basis are of great importance.

Many volunteers tend to come in at Thanksgiving, Christmas, and to have one more visit during the year, but this is not enough. It is important to see patients on a regular basis, and it is also important to schedule activities which are not just easy for the volunteer and for the nursing personnel in institutions but also pleasurable for the patient. It is advisable to go to the movies or to church away from the home if it is possible for the patient to do so. Visits away from the home with other people, for example, to golden-age centers or similar groups, should be encouraged. Taking the patient out of the family to see friends or acquaintances or to return to former haunts to which the patient was accustomed to going can be very therapeutic.

Family participation, where it is beneficial, can be vital. It is important never to cut ties completely. Even where conflict exists, with professional help some attempt can be made to resolve it. The patient upon returning home for a visit may react with a feeling of anxiety and agitation when reminded of what he once was. This risk is often worth the effort because there can be good effects if the family handles the patient's visit intelligently. Too often the family saves up ammunition for a shooting and shouting match when the patient returns home. Past wrongs and injustices may be dredged up in order to satisfy needs to punish and be punished. This can be avoided. It is probably just as important for the family to schedule activities for the patient's visit as it is for volunteers and for institutional personnel. Much of what was described above can be undertaken by family members.

Many resource groups are available in the community and can provide a catalog of activities which can be performed with patients, including arts and crafts activities using patients, sewing, knitting, crocheting, simple woodworking, and metal working. All these are possible. Again, it is much more important to determine the individual patient's personal interests and to establish a personal relationship with him. Concentration on the technical aspects of activities is misplaced. Ambitious vocational rehabilitation programs are inappropriate for this group. If a patient can do part-time work, it is certainly appropriate to assist him to do so. But to train him in new skills or to embark on ambitious rehabilitative programs is risky and may actually tend to be detrimental to the patients who are at a marginal level physically and mentally.

Deinstitutionalization can be fostered by organizing nursing care so that the patient who does not need twenty-four-hour care is not forced to accept it because nothing else is available. Thus day-care programs and night-care programs may be utilized. When patients are admitted to a hospital who can go home or to another setting for the night, day hospitalization is indicated. Clinic outpatient facilities for psychiatric treatment can help prevent or limit the duration of hospitalization. Barriers to the exchange of patients between hospitals and nursing homes, between homes for the aged and hospitals, and between the patient's own home and various institutions should be removed so that the patients can move freely without the administrative hurdles which are erected because of the inflexible policies and practices of many agencies. Communities should organize and integrate the services of various agencies around the patient rather than only around the agency. In this way patients do not get lost and go through a long period of screening followed by rejection because they do not meet the criteria for acceptance. Here again, guide lines are important, and agency personnel too often resist setting down their policies in a way which is easily interpretable by other people in the community.

Consultative services from institutions, particularly of a specialized kind, should be made available. The services of caseworkers, psychiatrically trained nurses, psychologists, as well as psychiatrists should be utilized when appropriate to assist in the evaluation and in the disposition of patients. Emergencies should be treated quickly. The family physician should have available to him the services of mental health personnel who can help him in planning and dealing with situations. It is the author's impression that many cases now being hospitalized could be kept at home if they were treated quickly during the acute phases of the crisis. Much of the problem lies in the fact that the general practitioner and family physician feel somewhat alone and relatively helpless in treating these disorders. If the services of psychiatric personnel and institutional services were available on a standby basis to family physicians, much of the harm of hospitalization could be avoided, and the length of hospitalization could certainly be cut down.

It is important to provide inservice training for family physicians so that they can recognize affective disorders. Quite often, depressions develop without too much notice taken of changes in the patients' mood. It is usually gradual, and it may manifest itself first with somatic symptoms and changes in activity level rather than in mood and in speech. It is important that these be recognized promptly and that treatment be instituted. Early hospitalization in some cases may result in marked improvement. The same is true for patients with senile brain disease. Some aspects of the latter are treatable if the patient is treated before deterioration has been allowed to proceed too far. In the very old there is a greater frequency in women than men because women live longer and have to be alone longer since they are widowed earlier. Perhaps a means can be found for handling these disorders in the family through treatment at home.

In spite of the irreversibility of chronic brain syndromes, some of the behavioral manifestations are treatable with carefully controlled dosages of tranquilizing medications or of antidepressants when appropriate. Some drugs such as ribonucleic acid, niacin, nicotine acid, PETN, and procaine have been claimed to be of value in treating the intellectual changes which go along with chronic brain syndrome. Evidence of their effectiveness is not consistent. Most recently, magnesium pemoline has been found to enhance acquisition and retention of a conditioned avoidance response in rats. This appears to be related to increased synthesis of brain nucleic acids. Clinical trials with humans are in process to determine its effect on learning and memory. For these agents, results are preliminary and await further validation.

Recent English studies show that there are many more aged patients who need help at home than in institutions. This is a challenge and also a threat because as medical facilities become available we can expect many more of these patients to seek hospitalization. The hospitals may very well be swamped by a sharp rise in admissions. Therefore, the criteria for admission to different facilities should be clearly delineated; for example, admission to geriatric hospitals, mental hospitals, nursing homes, homes for the aged, and rest homes.

One cannot end a section on psychiatric aspects of maintenance therapy of geriatric patients on a completely optimistic note. However, it should be noted that advances have been made and that there is an increased availability of community resources. With increased funds to become available in the ensuing years under Medicare, it is to be expected that facilities for the aged will increase in size and that quality of treatment will improve. Obviously there is a need for increased research in the area of pharmacological agents which might help reverse the progressive and irreversible deterioration in intellectual functions so basic to senile dementia. In general, treatment seems to be more effective in relation to situational crises, affective disorders, paranoid and schizophrenic disorders, as well as certain psychosomatic disorders. The best treatment from a psychiatric standpoint is one which makes use not only of pharmacological aids but also of psychological techniques. Of critical importance as well is the presence of a therapeutic environment. It is doubtful that any one agent or agents will be permanently helpful or curative without the presence of an environment which tends to encourage optimism and tends to support therapeutic action.

REFERENCES

1. WOLFF, K.: Group psychotherapy with geriatric patients in a mental hospital. *J. Amer. Geriatrics Soc.*, 5:13-19, 1957.
2. LINDER, M. E.: Group psychotherapy with institutionalized senile women.: II Study in gerontologic human relations. *Int. J. Group Psychother.*, 13:150-170, 1953.
3. HONIGFELD, G., ROSENBLUM, M. P., BLUMENTHOL, I. J., LAMBERT, H. L., and ROBERT, A. J.: Behavioral improvement in the older schizophrenic patient: Drug and social therapies. *J. Amer. Geriatrics Soc.*, 13:57-72, 1965.

Chapter VIII

MAINTENANCE THERAPY WITH DIABETIC PATIENTS

WILLIAM B. HADLEY

INTRODUCTION

SEVENTY-FIVE per cent of diabetes mellitus is discovered after the age of forty. With improved treatment of both diabetes and related or associated illness, a large percentage of these patients is living to age seventy and beyond. Mortality is steadily declining, and although it still exceeds that in the general population, the least excess is in older patients. When one adds to the above the frequently stated observation that diabetic patients become prematurely old, it is readily apparent that the care of the elderly diabetic is a major and steadily increasing problem.

Because diabetes is at present an incurable disease, it lends itself particularly well to the concept of maintenance therapy. Thus, all treatment is aimed at retarding or preventing progression of the disease and its complications. There is overwhelming evidence that such treatment does in most instances and in some degree accomplish this purpose. Steadily increasing longevity of the diabetic patient attests the effects of steadily improving treatment, the mainstays of which are education, diet, and either insulin or the oral compounds.

EDUCATION AND INSTRUCTION

Education and instruction of the patient and his relatives is an integral part of treatment of the diabetic patient. Diabetes is a way of life and must be approached from this viewpoint.

158

In many instances, care of diabetes in an elderly person becomes truly a family affair; this is particularly true where decreased vision, decreased hearing, or changes in mentation make adequate instruction of the patient impossible. All too often the elderly patient will procrastinate or conceal his symptoms for fear of causing expense to his family. In many instances it is the observant relative who insists on prompt medical attention. This is especially true with regard to care of the feet in the diabetic person with peripheral vascular disease or diminished pain sensation in the lower extremities. A responsible relative should be taught to examine the feet of the patient at a minimum of weekly intervals. White stockings should be worn so that the slightest amount of drainage from an otherwise unnoted lesion will not escape attention.

In the patient with peripheral vascular disease, pain is generally an important feature of accompanying necrosis or infection and in most instances brings prompt attention to the lesion. On the other hand, pain is generally absent or minimally present in the neuropathic foot, and extensive infection with osteomyelitis or microthrombosis and secondary necrosis is often present before medical attention is sought. The two major fears of the diabetic are loss of vision and loss of limb, and it is a paradox that procrastination because of fear of amputation frequently is responsible for progression of the disease to the point where amputation is necessary.

A large percentage of diabetic patients in the geriatric age group will have some degree of visual impairment, and a significant percentage of these will be legally blind (20/200 or less in Massachusetts). A blind or nearly blind patient poses particular problems in management, in large part related to his dependency on a relative or friend for the day-to-day care of his disease. He cannot test his urine, he cannot measure his insulin, and he cannot prepare and adhere to a diet. In addition to these rather obvious difficulties, the elderly blind patient is often depressed and actively or passively resists the efforts of others to help him. Although full rehabilitation is rarely possible in this age group, the patient should strive for a certain amount of independence which is consistent with health and safety. In almost all instances the patient can learn to walk with safety both in the house and out. All should be made aware of the many facilities, both private and governmental, which are available to the person without sight.

Careful instruction of the patient with regard to diet must be given, and the importance of regular testing of the urine must be emphasized. Perhaps most important is an understanding on the patient's part of the purposes of treatment. In most instances in this age group, diabetes is not symptomatic, and the importance of maintaining chemical rather than symptomatic control must be emphasized as a means of preventing later serious complications.

Certain general principles apply to treatment of the elderly diabetic. The majority of patients may be expected to respond quite satisfactorily to diet alone or to diet and one of the oral hypoglycemic agents. A very significant number, however, and this applies particularly to the individual with long duration of the disease or to those with abrupt, symptomatic onset, will require insulin. In general, when treatment other than just diet is required, one may expect this group of patients to be more sensitive to the effects of the particular drug than would be true in a younger population. The elderly person is relatively more fragile, lacks the resiliency of the younger person as regards various compensatory mechanisms in the body, and reacts poorly to overzealous use of many drugs including those employed in the treatment of the diabetes.

The major adverse effect of treatment is hypoglycemia. The brain is wholly dependent on glucose for its metabolism; and where cerebrovascular reserve is often already limited, the further effects on the central nervous system of insufficient glucose may be both frightening and serious. Treatment should be carefully individualized to avoid hypoglycemia and at the same time maintain a reasonable degree of control. In each instance the patient should be taught the signs and symptoms of hypoglycemia. In some instances the elderly person will fail to demonstrate or lack awareness of the early signs of hypoglycemia, and in such cases, compromise with the degree of control is a necessity. On the other hand, when hypoglycemic reactions are rare and are easily recognized, standards of control need not be relaxed. Hypoglycemic reactions are much less common with the oral agents than with insulin but do occur with overdosage and may be serious.

DIET

Diet is the cornerstone of therapy for the patient with adult-onset diabetes. It has been authoratively estimated that 70 per cent or more of this group of patients could be satisfactorily treated with diet alone were they willing to follow the necessary prescription to attain ideal body weight and maintain it. In practice, because symptoms are seldom present in sufficient degree to cause discomfort or annoyance, the majority of patients break their diets to greater or lesser degree. And yet, the diabetic diet is not a punitive one. The major restriction is in concentrated carbohydrate with lesser restriction in nonsweetened starches (bread, potato, macaroni, and so forth). Liberal protein is allowed to replace, in part, the reduction of carbohydrate. Fat is added to make up the total caloric prescription with emphasis today on adequate quantities of unsaturated fats.

Total caloric prescription is generally in the neighborhood of 25 to 30 calories per kg of weight. Daily carbohydrate seldom need exceed 150 gm and almost never 200 gm. This is in the form of fruit (1 oz. orange equals 3 gm); bread (1 oz. equals 15 gm); cereal (one oz. equals 20 gm); and vegetables, 20 per cent (potato, rice, corn, macaroni, and so on), 6 per cent (most yellow vegetables), and 3 per cent (most green, leafy vegetables). Milk cannot be overlooked, containing 1.5 gm carbohydrate per oz. Daily protein generally exceeds 60 but seldom 100 gm; common sources are meat, fowl, cheese, and fish. Thirty gm (1 oz.) meat contains 7; fowl, 8; cheese, 8; and fish, 6 gm protein. Amounts of fat are similar to those of protein, but because of the higher caloric value, fat often contributes double the quantity to total calories. Common sources are oil, butter, cream, cheese, meat, and nuts with 30-gm portions yielding 30, 25, 12, 10, 5, and 15 gm of fat respectively. The diet is best distributed through the day as three meals and either two or three small snacks at midpoints between meals or at bedtime.

The exchange diets sponsored by the American Diabetes Association, the American Dietetic Association, and the United States Public Health Service are readily available, easily learned, and quite accurate, provided that portions are measured. In teaching the diet the greatest emphasis should be placed on the fact that the diet is quantitative rather than qualitative. The patient should be encouraged to think not in terms of those foods which he may have or should avoid but rather in terms of the specific quantity of a particular food which he may have.

TREATMENT WITH THE ORAL COMPOUNDS

The majority of geriatric patients who fail to respond to dietary therapy alone will respond with the addition of one of the sulfonylureas or phenformin. It should be stressed from the beginning that these compounds do not replace but rather supplement a carefully followed dietary prescription. Duration of action is as follows: tolbutamide, 6 to 12 hr.; acetohexamide, 12 to 24 hr.; chlorpropamide, up to sixty hr. All apparently act primarily by stimulating release of insulin from pancreatic cells. Phenformin is available in either regular or timed release form; action is apparently through effects on peripheral glucose utilization and on the liver. There is no great difference in effectiveness between one and another of the above, and choice of compound is usually based on familiarity rather than specific advantage.

Treatment is begun usually with one tablet daily taken before breakfast, and the dose may be increased, if necessary, according to urine tests and blood sugars to that amount which provides either maximum effectiveness or unpleasant side effects. These amounts per day will be tolbutamide, 3 gm; acetohexamide, 1.5 gm; chlorpropamide, 0.5 gm; and phenformin, 150 to 200 mg. When switching from insulin to an oral agent, some advocate gradual substitution, but this is unnecessary provided that the patient is carefully followed. One should be particularly careful when considering the use of these compounds for patients of any age who have had grossly symptomatic onset of diabetes, have shown ketones in the urine at any time, or who require more than twenty units of insulin daily. A definite percentage of geriatric patients, perhaps more than 25 per cent, will be totally insulin dependent, lapsing into acidosis if insulin is discontinued.

Case Report

Mrs. M. B., age 68, diabetes known for twenty-two years. Initial onset was symptomatic with weight loss, polyuria, and polydipsia, and the patient had never been more than 10 per cent overweight. Diabetes had been moderately well controlled with six units of crystalline insulin mixed with twenty units of neutral protamine Hagedorn insulin each morning together with a 1,200-calorie exchange diet. Approximately one month prior to admission, the patient's regular physician had died, and she had seen a new physician who advised trial with tolbutamide. Insulin was gradually withdrawn, with tolbutamide being substituted over a period of one week's time. With 2 gm of tolbutamide daily on a carefully followed diet, urine tests before meals were mostly .5 to .75 per cent. The patient felt well and had no symptoms. Five days prior to admission the patient developed an upper respiratory infection and noted that urine tests were persistently 2 per cent for sugar. This continued for three days during which time the patient noted beginning of polyuria and polydipsia. Two days prior to admission the patient called her physician who advised increasing the dose of tolbutamide to three tablets, twice daily. Despite this change in dosage, symptoms continued, and one day prior to admission the patient noted increasing lethargy followed in succession by repeated vomiting, abdominal pain, and deep and rapid breathing. She was admitted to the hospital where a blood sugar was 720 mg per cent, with a carbon dioxide of 10 mEq liter and plasma acetone of 4+, 4+, 3+, 2+ in serial dilutions. The patient received a total of 320 units of insulin and five liters of intravenous fluid over a period of twelve hours and showed marked improvement.

Comment

Original symptomatic onset of diabetes, lack of obesity, duration of diabetes, and maintenance insulin dose of twenty-six units all argued against satisfactory response to sulfonylurea. In fact, response was only partial, resulting in asymptomatic but poorly controlled diabetes which was easily tipped over into a state of severe acidosis by intercurrent infection of a relatively minor type. A truly good response to oral compounds results in persistently sugar-free urine tests with generally better overall control of diabetes than can be accomplished with insulin. If such a response is not seen, the patient should be restarted on insulin.

INSULIN THERAPY

Insulin treatment is indicated for all geriatric patients who cannot maintain weight or adequate control of their diabetes by other means. The necessity for insulin treatment can be anticipated for those patients who present ketonuria or ketonemia and gross symptoms of weight loss, polyuria, and polydipsia. The normal or underweight patient will more often require insulin than the obese.

Types of Insulin
Types of Available Insulins

	Onset of Action (Hours)	Peak of Action (Hours)	Duration of Action (Hours)
Short			
Crystalline	1	2-4	6-8
Semilente	1½-2	5-7	12-18
Intermediate			
Globin	2-4	10-14	10-22
NPH (isophane)	1-2	10-20	20-32
Lente	1-2	14-18	26-30
Prolonged			
Protamine zinc	6-8	16-24	24-36
Ultralente	5-8	22-26	34-36

The initial dose of insulin is generally small, on the order of ten to sixteen units of intermediate-acting type. The dose is then adjusted in small increments until satisfactory control of blood and urine sugar is obtained. Initiation of treatment is generally accomplished in the hospital, where diet can be carefully controlled and proper provision made for instruction of the patient and his relatives. It must be understood that treatment of diabetes is a day-by-day proposition with regular urine tests forming a basis for adjustment of insulin dosage at specified intervals. In the older person, adjustment is generally made at three-day intervals, with persistent glycosuria during this period calling for an increase of two or more units. The before-supper test is the most reliable guide to the morning intermediate-acting insulin, with the test before lunch reflecting the amount of morning crystalline insulin. With protamine zinc insulin, the test before breakfast best reflects the previous day's dosage, and this same test is used to adjust the amount of intermediate-acting insulin which may, in some cases, be required at bedtime.

Diabetes is not a static disease, and some variation in the required amount of insulin can be anticipated over a period of weeks or months. Unusual stress such as infection or trauma may have a marked effect on requirement, and under these circumstances supplemental rapid-acting insulin (crystalline) may need to be employed. In general, supplemental crystalline insulin is given only when urine tests show persistent maximum reduction or particularly when ketonuria is present. The amount of crystalline insulin given under these circumstances is best related to the usual daily requirement with approximately one quarter to one third of the usual total daily dose being given in the form of crystalline at three-hour intervals according to urine tests. For example, the usual insulin dose equals ten crystalline plus thirty NPH given each morning; for consistently poor tests give $10+30=40x\frac{1}{4}=10$ units every three hours until test is less than maximum. In the presence of significant ketonuria $(4+)$ this amount may be increased by 50 per cent with fifteen rather than ten units being given under the same circumstances.

Intelligent use of insulin in this fashion plus an adequate fluid intake will obviate the necessity for hospitalization in a significant number of patients. In the presence of persistent vomiting or diarrhea, hospitalization is mandatory, but in most instances of acute illness, adequate fluid intake can be assured by regular, timed, small feedings. It is a dangerous but frequently accepted dictum that ketoacidosis rarely occurs in the geriatric age group. Actually a review of 401 cases of diabetic coma treated by physicians at the Joslin Clinic and the New England Deaconess Hospital between 1947 and 1961 revealed that 51 or 12.5 per cent were over sixty years of age at the time of admission. Mortality in this group was 11.8 per cent as compared to an over-all figure of 5 per cent for the entire group.

Insulin Hypoglycemia

As previously noted, the elderly patient tends to tolerate hypoglycemia poorly. Because of this, careful instruction must be given regarding the means of preventing its occurrence. Because of each type of insulin's particular activity curve, certain times of the day are particularly dangerous. With this in mind, special between-meal feedings are provided. Thus, with intermediate-acting insulins a midafternoon snack is provided, and a midmorning snack may be used to guard against hypoglycemia secondary to crystalline insulin. Unusual activity calls for special caution, and patients are instructed to take extra carbohydrate calories in order to anticipate and prevent low blood sugar at this time. In the case of patients in whom warning symptoms are lacking or poorly recognized, the family must be taught to be aware of and to treat such symptoms as sweating, tremulousness, mental confusion, or other unusual behavior.

Just as patients are taught to adjust their insulin dose upwards should urine tests show sugar, in a like manner they may be instructed to reduce the amount of insulin should urine tests be persistently sugar-free. In particular, they should not hesitate to reduce the amount of insulin materially (in the order of 10 per cent) should reactions occur without obvious cause. The most serious insulin reactions occur when insulin is given in the presence of already excessive insulin, and this circumstance most commonly occurs when no reduction is made after a series of minor reactions. In the final analysis most hypoglycemic episodes are iatrogenic and reflect lack of understanding on the part of the physician or inadequate instruction of the patient.

VASCULAR COMPLICATIONS

The major complications of diabetes mellitus are vascular. With increasing age, microvascular disease, as exemplified by diabetic nephropathy, plays a lessening role in morbidity, giving way to macrovascular disease involving the heart, brain, and peripheral vascular system.

Coronary heart disease is the major cause of death in diabetic patients, accounting for more than 50 per cent of total mortality. This compares with the figure of 30 per cent of all deaths in the United States in 1962 due to arteriosclerotic heart disease, including coronary artery disease. In living diabetic patients, depending upon the criteria used, the incidence of coronary heart disease varies from 20 to 40 per cent. In the diabetic, myocardial infarction often presents itself in an atypical fashion. Pain may be lacking in many instances or may occur in other than the usual location. Of particular importance is recognition of the fact that onset of congestive heart failure, unexplained nausea and vomiting, or sudden change in the behavior of the diabetic state may be the only clues to the occurrence of this serious complication.

Treatment of coronary artery disease in the diabetic in general follows the principles of management which apply to the non-diabetic. The patient with angina pectoris or the patient who has recovered from myocardial infarction is encouraged to be as physically active as his condition permits. Nitroglycerin is used freely for anginal pain or may be used prophylactically to prevent symptoms. The use of the longer-active coronary vasodilators is viewed with some skepticism, although in some instances they do seem to have a favorable effect. Anticoagulants are employed, if not contraindicated, in most cases of acute myocardial infarction where the diagnosis is made within forty-eight hours of the acute event or where congestive heart failure, shock, arhythmia, or thrombophlebitis is present. Long-term anticoagulation is generally not employed, and gradual withdrawal of the particular agent is most often accomplished between six to twelve months after infarction. Congestive heart failure is a common complication of coronary heart disease and is treated in the usual manner with sodium restriction, digitalis, diuretics, and limitation of activity.

Management of the diabetes itself usually poses no particular problem except in the immediate postinfarction period when intense hyperglycemia may be present with significant degree of insulin resistance. Much has been said about the risk of hypoglycemia in this group of patients, and fear of such complication may lead to neglect of reasonable standards of diabetic control. It is this author's experience that such fears are greatly exaggerated, and with careful attention to diet and insulin administration, good control can be maintained without frequent or severe episodes of hypoglycemia.

Cerebral vascular disease, which includes cerebral infarction and cerebral vascular insufficiency, is common among elderly diabetic patients, accounting for approximately 20 per cent of admissions to the New England Deaconess Hospital in the period of 1946-1957. Commonly, more than one if not all four major arterial trunks supplying the brain is involved. Infarction is often preceded by a period of recurrent episodes of insufficiency which may respond to conservative medical treatment. This consists of strict bed rest with the head level with or lower than the rest of the body, 5 or 10 per cent carbon dioxide inhalations to improve cerebral blood flow, control of postural hypotension when present, and gradual ambulation. With improvement in surgical methods for correcting cerebral insufficiency due to extracranial arterial lesions, careful evaluation of all four arterial trunks supplying the brain may be carried out by arteriographic techniques.

If infarction occurs, most often accompanied by hemiplegia or hemiparesis, physiotherapy is started early in the course of recovery and continued through the period of ambulation when this is possible. Because the period of recovery may be long, constant encouragement and expression of interest on the part of the physician and associated medical personnel may determine the success or failure of attempts at rehabilitation. In many diabetic cases there is small-vessel disease involving the brain as it does the eyes and kidneys. Such involvement, generally widespread, presents as dementia or arteriosclerotic parkinsonism.

Diabetic neuropathy, thought by many to be another manifestation of small-vessel disease through involvement of nutrient vessels to nerves, most commonly involves the sensory nerves, causing pain or paresthesias and sometimes dense anesthesia principally affecting the lower extremities. Motor involvement is less often seen and consists usually of a well-localized palsy involving one of the extraocular muscles with subsequent diplopia or the peroneal nerve with foot-drop.

Perhaps the most distressing type of neuropathy is that involving the autonomic nervous system. Postural hypotension may make standing or walking impossible but most often is a self-limited process responding to careful diabetic control and the use of 9-alpha-flurohydrocortisone. Lack of warning of hypoglycemic episodes due to interference with sympathetic and parasympathetic response may lead to sudden episodes of unconsciousness, sometimes with convulsions. Treatment consists of frequent, regularly spaced feedings and often compromise with the degree of control. Urinary or gastric retention due to an atonic bladder or stomach may interfere with proper nutrition and predispose to infection. Severe and refractory constipation due to neuropathic bowel involvement is very common in the diabetic and when accompanied by enforced bed rest for any reason may require regular enemas to prevent fecal impaction.

Peripheral vascular disease manifests itself in the diabetic as either arterial insufficiency or gangrene. Gangrene may result from gradual occlusion of main vessels without adequate development of collateral circulation. More commonly it occurs secondary to infection in the limb where marginal circulation has been maintained by collateral circulation. The most common underlying conditions leading to infection are fungus infection between the toes, paronychia, and dryness of the skin with fissure formation. The latter lesion is seen most commonly on the heel.

In the patient with marginal peripheral circulation, special care of the feet is mandatory and consists of regular podiatric attention to nails, corns, and callouses; the use of antifungual powder (such as Desenex®) between the toes; and the use of lanolin applied to the feet to prevent scaling and drying. White cotton stockings should be worn so that drainage or bleeding from an area on the foot will be noticed promptly. Treatment of an infected area consists of complete bed rest, appropriate antibiotics, debridement of dry necrotic tissue, and patience. Response to these measures will determine whether conservative therapy, local surgery, or an amputation will be necessary. Persistence of pain is an ominous sign. In some cases in which localized arterial blockage is present, reconstruction, resulting in improved blood flow to the foot and subsequent healing, may be possible.

When amputation is necessary, it may be performed at one of four levels. Simple removal of a toe is generally possible only in the presence of good circulation where either pedal pulses are present or excellent collateral circulation has been established below the knees. Transmetatarsal amputation is commonly employed at the New England Deaconess Hospital and at a few other centers but has not won widespread acceptance. Successful healing following this procedure leaves a reasonably good walking foot. When removal of the leg is necessary, the choice lies between below-the-knee and low-thigh procedures. Although healing is usually more prolonged, the former, when feasible, offers many advantages: walking with a prosthesis is easier and balance is better maintained either sitting or in bed, the incidence of persistent phantom limb pain is very low, and rehabilitation following leg amputation is successful in approximately two thirds of patients in the sense that a prosthesis is used. The majority of patients who do not walk again are limited by other medical illness, particularly coronary artery disease, congestive heart failure, or limited vision. Because of the generalized nature of vascular disease in the diabetic, approximately one half of those patients who have successful amputation of one extremity may be expected to develop some type of lesion on the opposite side, and approximately one third of these will go on to major amputation of the other extremity.

MAINTENANCE CARE

Because diabetes in the older person may often be associated with some degree of physical disability related to eye damage, peripheral vascular disease, cerebral vascular disease, or coronary thrombosis, many patients will require chronic maintenance care, most often in a nursing-home-type facility. For the most part, such care is less optimal principally because of lack of understanding, on the part of personnel, of the particular problems which beset this group of patients. Ideally, the transition from hospital to nursing home should be accomplished without interruption of the high level of specialized care which is obtained in the hospital. In fact, such is not the case and cannot be the case until closer liaison is established between the two types of facilities. With the increasing shortage of beds in acute care facilities there has been much discussion of the need for intermediate and long-term care facilities to allow more efficient utilization of acute bed space. In almost every hospital, average duration of stay could be materially shortened by having available adequate beds nearby so that intensity of treatment could be correlated with need. One can visualize the complete medical facility allowing optimal treatment on all levels of care under continuous integrated supervision.

There are numerous difficulties standing in the way of establishing such facilities, and not the least of these is cost. Adequate medical insurance coverage beyond the acute stage of illness has been a rarity. With the advent of Medicare, however, where provisions for continued convalescent and chronic care are an integral part of the program, such care may be offered to the geriatric patient on a financially self-sustaining basis. The same concept of integrated optimal-care facility is embodied in the program for cancer, stroke, and heart disease. Many feel that the nursing home can serve its proper purpose only as a satellite of the acute care hospital with both medical and administrative supervision integrated to provide maximum utilization.

At the present time, adequate care for the diabetic patient in a nursing home can be obtained only by personal supervision by a responsible physician at intervals dictated by the particular illness. In most cases, weekly visits will suffice provided that sufficiently clear and detailed orders are available for the nursing staff. In some instances, daily telephone communication may be necessary for the purposes of ordering insulin therapy for extremely unstable patients. Whatever the case may be, care of the diabetic patient with a recent stroke or heart attack can be anticipated to require somewhat more time and effort than the care of his nondiabetic counterpart, and it is the responsibility of the physician to see that this care is provided in an efficient but sympathetic manner.

The patient may regard the move to a nursing home as a

rejection by his children. In many instances the home represents the major tangible connection with the treasured past
whereas the nursing home represents the place of no return,
the final surrender, and a prelude to dying. Such a move is
usually easier for the elderly female as she accepts a passive
role with less feeling of sacrifice of independence. In the
case of the elderly man, however, retreat to a nursing home
implies withdrawal from an active adult role in life to a passive
childlike existence and may provoke various types of adjustments varying from withdrawal and increasing introspection
to greater self-assertiveness and belligerence as compensations
for feelings of insecurity.

In helping the patient to adjust to such an environment the
first resource is his relatives. They must be encouraged to
maintain contact by regular visits and indicate their interest
by serving as important members of the treatment group. In
many instances the physician can help to affirm this interest by
relaying advice and encouragement to the patient through one
of the family members. In every case, all efforts should be
made to convince the patient that he is not alone and forgotten
but is rather a focal point of care and interest.

One of the major problems in maintenance treatment of the
elderly diabetic is the fact that in this age group the majority
of patients have little symptomatology. Although there are
exceptions, as previously noted, in most instances the disease
is quite stable, and relatively gross evaluation in blood sugar
levels may lead only to such minor symptoms as fatigue, dry
mouth, muscle cramps, and occasional lightheadedness. Patients
tend to equate the state of control of their disease with the way
they feel rather than on the basis of urine or blood test results,
and constant emphasis must be placed on chemical rather than
symptomatic control as a means of preventing progression of
vascular disease.

The patient should be seen at intervals of from one to six
months depending on need, with the majority being followed
at intervals of three to four months. Complete physical examination should be done at least once yearly with laboratory studies
other than blood sugar and urinalysis being ordered as the

occasion demands. One must not forget that the diabetic is subject to other disease and that, in fact, most complaints requiring study and treatment will not be related directly to the level of blood sugar per se. Because proper treatment involves some sacrifice on the part of the patient, particularly in the area of dietary restriction, the physician must encourage, cajole, and, above all, explain again the necessity of following the program of treatment.

Many patients react to the discipline required in treatment by denying their disease. The insulin dose may be lowered without reason or in fact be completely omitted. Tests of the urine become less and less frequent particularly when they yield poor results as they remind the patient of his own inadequacy in dealing with his disease. Conversely, persistent sugar-free specimens may allow the susceptible patient to assure himself that there has been a mistake in diagnosis and that further treatment is unnecessary. The patient tends to believe only that which he wishes to believe; one should never use the term "mild diabetes" in discussion with a patient because "mild diabetes" soon becomes "no diabetes." The local street-corner medical expert is readily believed if his advice means an end to the unpleasantries of diet, regular urine tests, and expensive medicine. The patient who denies his disease is he who returns in ten years with complications involving the eyes, kidneys, and feet. "Treatment now for results in ten years" is the package which must be sold to the diabetic patient, and this is not considered a bargain by many.

Chapter IX

MAINTENANCE THERAPY FOR ARTHRITIC PATIENTS

WILLIAM H. CHASEN

IN DISCUSSING maintenance therapy for the chronic geriatric arthritic patient, one must deal with the most common varieties of arthritis, namely, hypertorphic osteoarthritis, rheumatoid arthritis, and gouty arthritis. Although there are numerous other forms of arthritis such as infectious, gonorrheal, luetic, tubercular, and so on, they are well controlled with antibiotics as well as antitubercular drugs. The only exception appears to be gonorrheal arthritis. Usually considered a disease of men, there is a rising incidence among men and women. Nevertheless, when a patient reaches the geriatric age, the diagnosis is usually well established.

Until two decades ago, arthritis was a disease with unknown etiology and indefinite treatment. However, in rheumatoid arthritis, the rheumatoid factor was identified. The rheumatoid factor is an abnormal autoantibody found in the blood of rheumatoid arthritis patients. It hooks on to gamma globulin and impairs its functioning. This rheumatoid factor can be found in patients with early rheumatoid arthritis by measuring levels of the rheumatoid factor. The severity and resultant deformities can be gauged by measuring rheumatoid factor levels.

The late Joseph Bunim, MD, of the National Institutes of Health, explained the presence of autoantibodies on the basis that the rheumatoid arthritic's immunological mechanism is deranged because of a genetic error. Dr. Bunim (1) believes that the normal body tissues has been altered by some noxious agent and that the immunological machinery does not recognize the altered cell as part of the body.

Gold therapy was first used in European countries beginning in 1911. It has a fairly high degree of undesirable side effects, with a 1 per cent mortality rate. With the advent of British anti-leuicite, mortality was cut to negligible proportions. In the Boston Veterans Administration Outpatient Clinic a series of fifty patients, with doses ranging from 10 to 50 mg weekly, had a very high proportion of proteinurias and dermatitis. When the medication was stopped, their conditions tended to clear, and when started again, they recurred. One cannot definitely say that any of these patients were helped with gold therapy.

With the advent of cortisone and adrenocorticotropic hormone by Kendall, and so on, in 1949 (2), new paths were opened. However, several side effects ensued with the use of the steroid hormones. There were also marked withdrawal reactions. The analogs permitted a lesser dose but no lesser side effects. Neither of these treatment methodologies solved the problem of rheumatoid or gouty arthritis and certainly had no effects on the degenerative joint diseases.

There are no known cures for chronic diseases. It is unlikely that one will ever be found for chronic arthritis. It is extremely difficult to imagine the medications which will reverse the changes in a chronic arthritic joint. Nevertheless, today drugs are available which when properly administered can control most forms of arthritis and gout. One of the most effective forms of therapy in the treatment of the chronic arthritic has been the use of physical therapy for which Dr. H. A. Rusk and E. G. Lowman (3) are primarily responsible. Following World War II, they spurred the developments in rehabilitation of all chronic diseases, particularly those in the geriatric group.

The spine is subjected to more stress than any joint in the body. Past the age of fifty, there is a great tendency for disc degeneration to occur. All forms of neck injury constitute a common cause of disc degeneration. Symptoms may be vague, with the principal complaint of numbness of the fingers, arms, or forearms. This may be accompanied by headaches. If there is pressure on the cord from spurs, the condition is known as spondylosis. Sayre traction and continuous use of the Thomas or cervical plastic collar will tend to alleviate the symptoms. Discography will help in the diagnosis.

When maintenance therapy is discussed, one must consider that the use of traction and the wearing of the cervical collar will become daily routine, and the patient must adjust to this condition. Patients in their sixty's and seventy's have managed to carry on useful occupations although wearing the collar constantly. Motivation is usually the determining factor between success and failure in the rehabilitation of all arthritic patients.

Calabro (4) gave an excellent summary in the management of ankylosing spondylitis. During the mid 1940's and early 1950's in the Veterans Administration Outpatient Clinic, Boston, Massachusetts, ankylosing spondylitis was treated with gold therapy and subsequently with x-radiation. Although there were many glowing reports in the use of gold therapy, very little success was achieved with this form of treatment. With x-ray therapy the average dose was 100 roentgens, usually for a total of 1,000 R. Relief lasting from several months to several years was obtained in at least 80 per cent of all patients. This procedure was abandoned because of the numerous reports that this type of therapy increased the incidence of leukemia. A twelve-year follow-up on patients treated in our clinic revealed that none developed any form of leukemia or other blood dyscrasias. Should a patient past the age of fifty be afflicted with distressful ankylosing spondylitis, x-radiation to the spine would be administered without hesitation. The questionable onset of leukemia would probably not occur until after the normal life expectancy of the patients. There still remains a question as to whether ankylosing spondylitis is a manifestation of rheumatoid arthritis or a separate disease.

Dr. Hans Waine and the author (5) studied approximately twenty-five patients with ankylosing spondylitis. For 80 per cent the latex fixation tests were negative; but for the 80 per cent the latex inhibition tests were positive, a result which certainly does not rule out rheumatoid disease. The sedimentation rate is invariably elevated. With very few exceptions, ankylosing and spondylitis begins with low back pain, morning stiffness, and limited back motions. Approximately one fourth of all ankylosing spondylitis will go on to involvement of both hips; of these, one half will have permanent destruction necessitating bilateral cup arthroplasty or insertion of an artificial head and neck. These procedures eventually break down, and the spondylitic thus involved usually does not live long enough to become a geriatric patient. Where there is no hip involvement, there may be moderate to marked kyphoscoliosis. Where marked, there may occur aortic insufficiency and early death. If the patient with (ankylosing spondylitis) is well motivated, he may attain a ripe old age with minimal deformity. This rests primarily on his desire and capacity to do the proper exercises daily, seven days a week, throughout his lifetime.

Patients are cautioned that exercises must be stopped immediately at the first sign of pain or tiredness. This is essential if joint destruction is to be prevented. The use of steroid hormones can become hazardous because the patient, unaware of pain, may abuse his joints by overuse with resultant destruction. Exercises are started minimally and gradually increased to approximately fifteen to twenty minutes per day. It may take thirty to sixty days to achieve this result. The disease usually progresses to involve the entire spine as well as the symphysis pubis and chest wall with restricted chest expansion. The chest weight exercises performed by patients at the Boston Veterans Administration Outpatient Clinic increased chest expansion of some of the patients from as little as one quarter of an inch to two inches in a period of four to eight weeks.

Systematic manifestations of ankylosing spondylitis are similar to those of peripheral rheumatoid arthritis, namely, weight loss, anemia, mild fever, early fatigue, and iritis. Several of the patients at the Boston VA Outpatient Clinic developed amyloydosis and cardiac involvement. These were noted in patients who had a strong desire to maintain their disease in the deformed state. Psoriasis, ulcerative colitis, and Reiter's syndrome occurred fairly frequently in ankylosing spondylitis as they do in peripheral rheumatoid disease.

In the treatment of ankylosing spondylitis, the use of hot baths for a period of twenty minutes at bedtime, and twenty-five grains of aspirin, three to four times per day, is advised; these help to relieve pain and spasm. Should ringing in the ears occur, the dosage is gradually diminished to tolerance. Indocin® has been found of value, but one half of the patients developed marked headaches or gastrointestinal disturbances. The patients were given two tablets twice daily. Some were subsequently cut to one tablet three times a day, one tablet twice a day, and one tablet daily, with equal therapeutic effect. The possible placebo effect of this drug is still to be evaluated.

Of all the arthritides, gouty arthritis is the most amenable to therapy. For the past twelve years, by the use of uricosuric agents such as Benemid® and Anturane®, acute attacks have been allayed. Most of the acute exacerbations are readily controlled with colchicine—one every hour until toxic manifestations such as nausea, vomiting and/or diarrhea occurred. Phenylbutazone—200 mg four times a day the first day and 200 mg three times a day the second day—will usually cause an acute flare-up of gout to subside. In the Outpatient Clinic, allopurinal, a xanthine oxidase inhibitor, is also used and shows great promise of containing the acute exacerbations of gout. Not infrequently, patients with gout also have rheumatoid disease as well as hypertrophic arthritis. This possibility must be considered in the over-all therapy of the geriatric arthritic.

One cannot overstress the importance of the psychiatric evaluation of the arthritic since emotional concomitants are a vital stress factor. Listening to all the patient's complaints including his home environment, attitude of his family, nursing care, entertainment, and so on offers reassurance and helps to reduce anxiety. If he is not integrated into his home life, he may become depressed. In some instances, mental confusion occurred and these patients were referred to psychiatric hospitals. Social workers are invaluable in assessing the psychological conditions of arthritics and providing casework services essential to maintenance. Newer psychiatric therapies, especially psychotherapy and the use of tranquilizers in combination with the physical and chemical maintenance measures, has led to the rehabilitation of many arthritic patients. The ability to perform useful functions enhances their self-esteem.

With a small grant from the Arthritis Foundation the physical therapy department at the Boston Veterans Administration started an occupational therapy unit including work-compensated therapy activities. As maintenance therapy, this program has been invaluable because of its psychological impact in developing constructive attitudes of well-being. It has also enabled some arthritics to make use of their deformed fingers in a useful endeavor as well as preventing ankylosis and further deformities. It is amazing how well geriatric patients can function with deformities after having received physical therapy and the use of proper exercises in rehabilitation programs.

Motivation in one of the most important factors in the prevention of deformity in rheumatoid arthritic patients. It is surprising how many resist therapy and allow deformities to develop. Thus, instead of alleviation, their condition worsens. There are several striking examples which will illustrate this phenomenon.

CASE HISTORIES

Case 1

A patient who was in practice with his brother in a related medical field came to the Clinic in 1950 with moderate dorsal kyphosis and beginning fusion of the spinal ligaments. He was placed on a course of steroid hormone therapy plus exercises and became symptom-free with an excellent posture. Because of certain psychological factors, he also was unhappy. He did not report to the Clinic and for two and one half years stopped all his medication and exercises. When he returned, taken by his brother by the hand like a small boy, he was severely deformed. Now that he was permanently deformed, he seemed to be content as long as his brother and others hovered over him.

Case 2

In 1950 a married female in her early thirties came to the Veterans Administration Outpatient Clinic with typical ankylosing spondylitis. She had moderate dorsal kyphosis, secondary anemia, weight loss and typical x-ray changes. After a short course of steroid hormone therapy, her spine straightened, her anemia was no longer present, and her weight was normal for age and height. This was one of the most satisfying results of steriod therapy any physician could desire. For some reason she became depressed, stopped the prescribed exercises, and refused to report for treatment. She returned eighteen months later with marked kyphotic deformity, moderate anemia and weight loss, but she was also less depressed and appeared more contented with her lot. A psychiatric consultation revealed that she was in constant fear of losing her husband and was convinced that the only way to keep him was to maintain her deformed state. The fact that she also received 100 per cent Veterans Administration disability pension was perhaps an additional motivating factor. At present she also has amyloid disease. Psychiatric treatment was attempted for several years but resulted in failure.

Case 3

A surgeon requested that the author examine his older brother, age fifty-six, who had ankylosing spondylitis with three-inch shortening of one leg. He was markedly kyphotic and had a built-up shoe. He had severe pain over the entire spine. A detailed history revealed that his father was a well-known physician whose desire was to have the eldest son follow in his footsteps. The son had no interest in medicine and soon developed symptoms of spondylitis. Although he received expert medical care, he continued to develop a kyphotic deformity including destructive changes in the left hip resulting in a three-inch shortening. He evidently had a burn-out spondylitis, and laboratory studies revealed an elevated uric acid. Treatment with colchicine and Benemid resulted in control of his symptoms. His brother was anxious to have his kyphotic deformity corrected. When this was suggested the patient became panicky. It was further elicited that his deformity gave him a certain status. His neighbors admired him because he could lift a sixty pound sack despite his deformity. He also fathered five children although he married at age fifty. At church and social gatherings he was admired for his stamina. One can readily imagine that if he lost his deformity he would lose his social status which gave him a great deal of security and satisfaction.

These patients are not rare exceptions but rather common. A person with rheumatoid arthritis, if properly motivated, can in most instances prevent deformity, but it takes a great deal of effort. Without proper motivation, treatment is bound to fail.

For the past decade, phenylbutazone has been used for short-term therapy with marked beneficial effects. However, phenylbutazone is known to have caused blood dyscrasias as well as activation of peptic ulcers. In recent months, Indocin has been used which, although effective, has tended to give undesirable side reactions such as severe headaches and gastrointestinal reactions. These symptoms subsided with lessening of the doage.

Dr. L. Sullivan (6) reported that latent infections has been activated in patients undergoing Indocin therapy. In one patient a hip infection was brought to light; aseptic arthritis was reactivated. In three others the contention was that indomethacin does not cause a reduction in antibody formation and that it is possible that activation of local infection is due to a breakdown of local barriers to the spread of infection. Merck, Sharp and Dohme* stated that this consequence was merely coincidental, since their study of the drug with pre-infected animals demonstrated no effect on the course of preexisting infection—which was not true of the steroids.

Recently, dimethyl sulfoxide has received a great deal of publicity. Used locally as a liniment it was reported to have given marked relief to the area applied. This drug was withdrawn by the Federal Food and Drug Administration because of changes in the refractive index of lenses of experimental animals. Others have reported tissue destruction. Impaired circulation caused by red cell clumps in the capillary beds and coating of the arterioles was thought to be responsible for the damage when it was used as an antineoplastic agent. Dr. Joseph B. Sarner of the University of Pennsylvania School of Medicine (7) reported the use of 10 cc of 90 per cent solution in water applied to the sacrococcygeal areas on an obsorbent cotton sponge gave relief in five to ten minutes, permitting manipulation of the bone and its attachments. A single preparation gave relief from five to seven hours. There was local pruritis after treatment which was self-limited with no residuals. Dr. Jack Zuckner of the St. Louis University School of Medicine (8) gave DMSO alone and in combination with a steroid compound (1 per cent triamcinolone actetonide). Dimethyl sulfoxide was applied over inflamed joints four times daily. The treated area was covered five times with each application for a period of ten days.

In treatment with DMSO of post-traumatic soft tissue injuries

---

*A drug company.

to the upper or lower spine, there have occurred strains of the larger joints of the extremities, acute post-traumatic soft tissue injuries associated with subcutaneous and intramuscular bleeding of the trunk or extremities, and acute bursitis as well as gout effecting the larger bone joints. Dr. J. Harold Brown of Seattle (9) reported 85 per cent had good to excellent results on treatment with an 80 per cent solution. Ninety-four per cent had good to excellent results on a 60 per cent solution. Use of the 90 per cent solution brought good to excellent results in 84 per cent, but one third had to discontinue treatment because of side effects. Eight to 12 cc of DMSO solution was applied by the patient or a member of the family over a wide area circumscribing the affected joint. Dr. P. L. Day of the University of Texas School of Medicine (10) studied 970 patients and reported good to excellent results in 847: 365 patients with arthritis; 71 of 141 with bursitis; and 74 of 120 with acute trauma, as well as low back pain and gout. Half of the patients had transient or localized dematitis controlled with bland ointments or change in dosage; 170 discontinued the drug because of side effects.

Dr. Arthur Steinberg of the Albert Einstein Medical Center, Philadelphia (11), treated over one hundred patients with musculoskeletal disorders and claimed a favorable response in 80 per cent. Best results were in acute tendinomusculoskeletal disorders. He claimed no serious side effects. Dr. Arthur Ruskin of the FDA (12) pointed out that there were no properly controlled trials—only many testimonials.

Self-help devices (13) have been designed to permit various deformed joints to function and thus render the patient self-sufficient. Many devices have been developed to enable the patient to function despite severe deforming arthritis. Now available are aids to feeding and getting in and out of a bed, or car by various canvas slings and hydraulic devices which enable these patients to function with minimal help. Some devices enable the patient to help himself with minimal effort such as safety grips on bathtubs, devices for lathering with soap, combing hair, clipping nails, dressing, and reaching for objects as well as picking up food and turning pages of a book. There are also designed appliances for the knees, back, and feet, as well as for keeping the posture correct.

Probably the single most important treatment for the chronic geriatric arthritic is the proper use of physical exercises. It is helpful to outline a definite program of exercises, some of which may be accomplished at home. Hydrotherapy such as the use of the Hubbard tanks, whirlpool baths, ultrasound, diathermy, and hydrocollators are invaluable adjuncts to therapeutic exercises in treating the severely deformed arthritic.

EXERCISES

Spinal and Cervical Exercises

Exercises are necessary to keep the spine as flexible as practicable. The patient first tries out various maneuvers under supervision in the Clinic where he is also cautioned that no exercise is to be continued past the point of pain or fatigue. The exercises which are taught at the Clinic may be done for only one or two minutes at the start, but they are gradually increased to ten or twelve minutes: This usually takes about one month.

In the Clinic's Physical Medicine Section, many patients with cervical arthritis—and such cases are numerous—are given Sayre traction using weights ranging from five to fifteen pounds. The use of a plastic cervical collar is advisable, and most patients manage to sleep while wearing it.

Upper Extremity Exercises

For finger exercise, the use of a small rubber ball squeezed several times a day for one to three minutes at a time, if possible, has been found to be very useful. This is best done underwater while the patient sits in a hot tub. When the hands are very painful, hot wax is used, followed by finger exercises such as using the rubber ball and picking up various-sized coins or similar objects. Elbow exercises are accomplished by ball throwing—extending and flexing the elbow and raising the arms above the head.

It is necessary to rule out acute bursitis before prescribing any shoulder exercises. If an acute bursitis is present, the most useful procedure has been the intramuscular injection of ACTH gel,

1 cc (40 international units) daily for two to three days, provided that there are no contraindications such as diabetes, hypertension, or peptic ulcer. When the acute attack subsides, shoulder exercises may be resumed with traction of the arms performed by the physical therapist. A good shoulder exercise is moving an imaginary wheel (at the side of a wall) in a rotary motion, followed by raising and lowering the arm.

In the chronic phase of rheumatoid arthritis, in which surgery was not accomplished and the progression of the disease has been severe enough to damage articular surfaces, arthrodesis of one or several joints may be helpful in relieving pain, establishing stability, and improving function. According to Dr. J. Leonard Goldner of the Duke University School of Medicine (14), excision of the greater multangular bone at the base of the thumb as part of an arthroplasty frequently helps to maintain motion and diminish pain. A normal joint is never obtained after surgery, but pain is lessened and the rate of progressive change is decreased.

Early surgery is much preferred to late salvage. Nevertheless, prior to any surgery, the patient should have good medical management and be motivated to receive surgical reconstruction. Rheumatoid arthritis starts as a synovitis with marked proliferation of the synovium. Early removal of the synovium will prevent destruction of ligaments and articular cartilage by pannus formation, as well as prevent destruction of the subchondral bone. According to Dr. Leonard Marmor of the University of California, Los Angeles School of Medicine (15), a new synovium which is not rheumatoid will regenerate in three to four weeks. Patients who have had a synovectomy and have exacerbation of the rheumatoid arthritis at a later date do not suffer from swelling or pain in the joints which were operated on.

Dr. Paul R. Lipscomb of the Mayo Clinic (16) maintains that it is usually impractical to perform surgery on all rheumatoid joints. Nevertheless, the wrists and small joints of the hands, particularly the metacarpophalangeal and proximal interphalangeal joints can be treated by surgical synovectomy. Excision of the distal end of the ulna, which is loosened or disconnected early in rheumatoid arthritis, is necessary when performing synovectomy of the wrist and will also prevent rupture of the extensor tendons later.

The chief complication of early or late surgery in all patients with rheumatoid arthritis is stiffness. Supervised activities and proper use of splints will help to prevent this stiffness to a great extent. Before considering surgery, immobilization by casts, gentle exercises, and when indicated, aspiration of fluid plus local hydrocortisone should first be attempted. If this fails, total excision of the involved synovial sheath is good prophylactic treatment. It must be kept in mind that rheumatoid arthritis is a progressive disease, and unless controlled by maintenance therapy, all surgery will result in failure.

It is rarely necessary for geriatric patients with rheumatoid arthritis to receive steroid therapy. It should be administered only in severe, acute exacerbations and then only when simpler methods fail. In any event, steroid therapy should be kept to a minimum. It should be particularly avoided in patients who have a drug dependency. When steroid therapy is used, it is best to give it on alternate days or in combination with another immunosuppressive agent. Harter *et al.* (17) showed that when patients on steroid therapy were given twice the daily dosage every other day in a single dose, the hypothalamic-pituitary-adrenal reserve function was better maintained; undesirable effects on supporting tissues such as bone, skin, and connective tissue were lessened; and termination of treatment was made easier. Local administration of corticosteroids has a minimum of undesirable, generalized effects. Since many geriatric patients have osteoporosis, and the condition is enhanced with steroid treatment, extra caution should be used with x-rays before the start of treatment. Prior to starting on steroids administration there should be an evaluation of the pituitary-adrenal status, appropriate tests of carbohydrate metabolism, x-ray films of chest and spine, ECG, upper GI series in patients with history of peptic ulcer, and evaluation of the patient's psychological status.

Oral steroids are best used in long-term adrenocorticoid treatment, and ACTH is reserved for activating the adrenal cortex before final withdrawal of corticosteroids. Adrenocorticotropic hormone therapy induces greater salt and water retention than with synthetic glucocorticoid. For the past twelve years, ACTH gel, 1 cc intramuscular (40 international units), was used for all cases of acute bursitis with excellent results. The average dose was 1 cc, IM, daily for three successive days. This should be avoided in patients with diabetes mellitus, coronary disease, and patients with histories of peptic ulcers or hypertension. Local steroid or 1 cc hydrocortisone may be injected locally in the involved joint of ACTH treatment is contraindicated.

SUMMARY

In this chapter the significance of maintenance therapy for the arthritic patient has been discussed. It was stressed that although chronic arthritis is not a curable condition, if proper maintenance measures as prescribed by the physician are carried out, the patient can lead a useful life with minimal deformity. Maintenance therapy procedures which were described included chemotherapy, psychiatric treatment, surgical reconstruction, physical medicine, and rehabilitation.

REFERENCES

1. BUNIM, J.: Academy of Medicine. *New Jersey Bull.*, 9:39-51, 1963.
2. KENDALL, E. C.: Collected papers. *Mayo Clin. Proc.*, 42:8, 1950.
3. LOWMAN, E. G.: *Arthritis*. Boston, Little, 1959.
4. CALABRO: *Bull. Rheum. Dis.*, April, 1966.
5. WAINE, H., and CHASEN, W.: In publication.
6. SULLIVAN, L.: *Medical Bulletin*, 1966.
7. SARNER, J. B.: *Medical Bulletin*, 1965.
8. ZUCKNER, J.: Intramuscular administration of steroids in treatment of rheumatoid arthritis. *Ann. Rheum. Dis.*, 23:456-462, 1964.
9. BROWN, J. H.: *Medical Tribune* (conference report), March 30, 1966.
10. DAY, P. L.: *Medical Tribune* (conference report), March 30, 1966.
11. STEINBERG, A.: *Medical Tribune* (conference report), March 30, 1966.
12. RUSKIN, A.: *Medical Tribune* (conference report), March, 1966.
13. Self-Help Devices. Arthritis Foundation, 10 Columbus Circle, New York, New York.
14. GOLDNER, J. L.: *Medical Tribune* (conference report), January 29-30, 1966.
15. MARMOR, L.: *Median nerve compression in rheumatoid arthritis.*
16. LIPSCOMB, P. R.: *Proceedings* 40:132-164 (53 references) 1965.
17. HARTER, *et al.*: Surgery of arthritic hand. *Brit. Med. J.*, 5441:1065, 1965.

Chapter X

MAINTENANCE THERAPY IN VISION AND HEARING FOR GERIATRIC PATIENTS

BENJAMIN BELL

VISION

THIS chapter is written for the people who have some responsibility in keeping an aging person functioning, for
example, rehabilitation and nursing home personnel. Material
is also included of practical value for general physicians, who
have more frequent and available contact with the geriatric
patient than the specialist in eye diseases.

Normal Structures

Protective Structures

The eye is contained in a protective bony cage called the
orbit and is also surrounded by protective soft tissues, of which
the lids or palpebra constitute the front boundary. The lids are
lined by a fine membrane called the palpebral conjunctiva,
which extends over the white of the eye where it is called the
bulbar conjunctiva. The lids contain skin glands which secrete
at the margins of the lids, hair follicles from which the lashes
grow, and the opening of the tear canals.

Coats of the Eye

The eye has an outer protective coat which is called the sclera
and contains an opening in the back for the optic nerve and
blood vessels. The sclera forms the visible white of the eye which
ends at the margin (limbus) of the cornea or transparent window
of the eye. Visible through the cornea is the pigmented iris diaphragm which has continuity with the middle coat of the eye
called the choroid. The innermost coat of the eye is the retina,

whose nerve fibers from the optic nerve conducting the visual impulses to the brain where images are perceived. The small area of the retina responsible for central or straight-head vision is called the macula. The macula area is responsible for the fine discriminative function involved in reading. If one charts the visual fields, a defect in this region produces a blind spot called a central scotoma. This is not to be confused with the normal or physiological blind spot which corresponds with the disc formed by the optic nerve. Between the optic disc and the macula there is an arching bundle of nerve fibers. The retina extends peripherally to the equator and from there anteriorly to the serrated border which is the ora serrata. The blood vessles of the retina consist of the central artery and vein which pass through the optic disc and branch into smaller vessels called arterioles and venules.

Transparent Media of the Eye

Light is transmitted to the retina through normally transparent structures, called the transparent or refractive media, namely, the cornea, the aqueous fluid, the lens, and the vitreous body, in the order named going from the front to the back of the eye. The cornea and a small overhang of the sclera in front, and the iris and central part of the lens in the back, form a dome-shaped chamber (the anterior chamber) which contains a clear fluid (aqueous). The fluid is formed by a structure called the ciliary body, which is contiguous with the root of the iris. The fluid drains out through a filtration system in the angle of this chamber. The lens is supported by zonular fibers so that the front of it is in the plane of the iris. The lens receives light according to the size of the iris diaphragm and focuses it on the retina by the action of the ciliary muscle which is capable of changing the shape of the lens. The vitreous or glassy body, a gellike structure, occupies the large space behind the lens and in front of the retina.

Examination of the Eye

External

The external examination of the eye may be performed by a focused light beam (focal illumination). Introduced obliquely in the form of a slit, an optical section of the transparent media is visualized, which may be studied in detail by means of loupe magnification in the hand slit lamp or by miscroscopy in the stationary instrument.

Internal

The interior of the eye can be illuminated and visualized simultaneously by an ophthalmoscope. In the ophthalmoscopic picture we actually see living columns of blood and a disc of living nerve tissue. The retinal vascular system consists of gracefully contoured arteries and veins, whose caliber bear an approximate ratio of two to three, and which emerge and converge respectively at the optic disc. The central retinal artery may have its primary division either in the substance of the optic nerve, or on the surface of the disc. The secondary division results in the formation of the superior and inferior temporal and nasal arteries. Peripheral to this, the vessels are of the caliber of arterioles. The tributaries of the veins follow the same general course as the arterial branches. The central retinal vein leaves the globe in the substance of the optic nerve. The optic nerve, made up of central processes of the ganglion cells of the retina, leaves the globe through a canal in the sclera 1.5 mm in diameter. The coats of the optic nerve are continuous with the corresponding coats of the brain and end blindly on the sclera. Only the intraocular portion of the optic nerve, called the nerve head or optic disc, is visible ophthalmoscopically, although changes in the retrobulbar portion may be reflected in the visible part.

General Decline of Visual Function in Aging

The pupils get smaller, and the refractive media, notably the lens, become less transparent, resulting in diminished illumination of the retina. At the same time there is less tolerance to glare, so that at the time of life when the patient needs more light to see and to read well, he can tolerate bright light less. Accordingly, lighting with optimal illumination on the visualized material, with minimal glare, must be provided for these patients. The lens also loses capacity to accommodate or focus objects clearly on the retina, requiring careful refraction and proper spectacles to compensate for this accommodative loss, and for the tendency of the lens cortex to enlarge with age. Indeed, the nucleus of the lens hardens (nuclear sclerosis) with age, attaining compactness to offset this cortical enlargement.

Local Eye Diseases

Protective Soft Tissues

The protective soft tissues undergo changes resulting in improper apposition of palpebral and bulbar conjunctive, with impaired lacrimal function, impingement of cilia on the cornea, or both. It follows that the cornea exposed in the palpebral aperture will require protection in maintenance therapy including appropriate topical medication, local compresses, and epilation of the offending lashes by cilia forceps, with the aid of loupe magnification; and referral for surgical intervention in severe cases of inversion or eversion of the lids, skin folds which hang over the palpebral fissure, overgrowths of the bulbar conjunctive onto the cornea, lachrymal duct obstruction, and retention cysts of the lids.

Cornea

The cornea is also subject to senile degenerative processes, the most common and best known being the innocuous arcus senilis. Other peripheral corneal changes likewise do not affect vision unless extension to the central part of the cornea occurs. A slit lamp examination of the cornea accordingly becomes an important part of the periodic eye examination in older patients. Although the stationary slit lamp and microscopic combination available in specialists' offices and in eye clinics is the instrument of choice, a hand slit lamp or a Barkan illuminator will provide adequate focal illumination for diagnostic purposes in the home or by the nonspecialist if used in combination with magnification such as the Beebe loupe.

Lens

The lens may manifest demonstrable changes which are completely asymptomatic and visible only as spokes in the periphery under dilation of the pupil. Nevertheless, as any lenticular opacity, they are called cataracts. Accordingly, a cortical cataract which interferes with vision is a late manifestation of an earlier process. Similarly, a senile nuclear cataract is a late manifestation of ongoing nuclear sclerosis. Some older people will not have vision-impairing cataracts which interfere with their needs and activities within their life span. A large number will, and can look forward to restoration of adequate vision by generally safe and successful surgical intervention in which the lens of the more impaired eye is usually extracted first. The other cataract may be removed at a later date. Maintenance therapy will depend on the post operative fitting of the aphakic eye with proper spectacles to achieve maximal monocular vision, or even binocular single vision by means of contact lenses. The latter requires a highly motivated and cooperative individual who is physically able to handle these lenses safely and effectively. In either case, interpretation and counseling is an important part of the regimen. Even though the patient has had a successful restoration to normal vision, he must understand the limitations imposed by the corrected aphakia as compared to the normally phakic eye. This is particularly important during the period when the patient is adjusting to his eyeglasses and has not yet become accustomed to the magnification effect and to the readjustment of eye-hand coordination.

Vitreous

The vitreous may undergo primary degenerative changes which may be manifest to the patient as floating bodies in the field of vision and dismissed as innocuous. On the other hand, involvement of the vitreous may be secondary to more serious diseases involving the retina. Accordingly, the consciousness of such floating bodies, with or without disturbing aberrant light phenomena, merits a prompt and thorough evaluation of the retina.

Retina

The retina is subject to central retinopathy easily seen by ordinary direct ophthalmoscopy and called senile macular degeneration, and to peripheral degenerative changes whose adequate visualization requires skilled binocular indirect ophthalmoscopy with scleral depression. The former is a common cause of reduced visual acuity and the discrimination required in comfortable reading, and of disappointment in attaining adequate vision after cataract operation. The latter is an inadequately explored no-man's-land because of the high degree of technical skill and knowledge involved in its meaningful visualization which up to now has been principally used in retinal detachment charting and in the detection of predetachment lesions. The development of more-sensitive peripheral field testing may throw more light on this area between the equator and the ora serrata. There should be a correspondence between abnormalities in the periphery and studies on retinal sensitivity.

Glaucoma

Glaucoma is the local eye disease which destroys vision by its pressure effect on the optic nerve head. The acute angle-closure or congestive type constitutes a curable surgical emergency, whereas the open-angle or so-called chronic simple type requires maintenance therapy. The physician who has assumed the health and functional maintenance of the geriatric patient, often a generalist, should be able to recognize both types. To accomplish this it is desirable that he have a record of a complete ophthalmological examination which includes a gonioscopic evaluation of the status of the anterior chamber filtration angle, namely, whether it is easily closable by apposition of the iris to the outer wall of this angle because of its narrow configuration or the presence of adhesive processes, or whether it will remain open even when the pupil is dilated. In many cases the nonspecialist can estimate this for himself by use of the handslit lamp with magnification as previously mentioned.

The oblique illumination will project the slit image on both the surface of the iris and on the cornea. As these simultaneous images are swept from the center to the limbus, an estimate as to whether there is a shallow anterior chamber and narrow angle, or a deeper chamber and a wide angle, can be made. The former may develop an acute closure with pain and congestion resembling an acute inflammation except that the eye is hard and the pupil dilated. The latter may be painless and insidious in its course. The acute type demands immediate treatment to conserve vision and is in fact curable by a simple peripheral iridectomy, to relieve the pupillary block.

If specialized assistance is not promptly available, the generalist may employ hyperosmotic agents such as 50 per cent glycerine by mouth (1 cc per pound of body weight). While waiting for specialized help, this will in fact enable the ophthalmic surgeon to operate more promptly because a reduction in tension is desirable before the operative procedure, and the surgeon usually accomplishes this by the use of miotics locally and hyperosmotic agents (mannitol, urea) systemically, as well as by acetazolamide (carbonic anhydrase inhibitor), in order to perform the iridectomy on a quiescent eye.

The maintenance therapy of the open-angle type requires that the physician be versed in the use of the Schiotz's tonometer, the ophthalmoscope, and the tangent screen. The use of the tonometer requires the instillation of anesthetic drops, is easily tolerated by the patient, and easily mastered by the physician. The ophthalmoscope will reveal the state of the optic nerve head, and the progression of excavation and atrophy is visualized by the dipping of the vessels over the rim of the disc. In severe cupping with undermining of the disc margin, the vessels will disappear at the disc margin and reappear in the center of the cup. The tangent screen using the one-millimeter white test object at a distance of one meter enables charting of the field to an isopter of thirty degrees. Thus, increase in size of the blind spot and development of the characteristic arcuate scotomata extending nasally from the blind spot to form a typical nasal step, can be readily determined.

Using the same test object at a distance of two meters, the temporal field normally passes just outside the blind spot. Accordingly, a slight loss in the temporal field will merge with the blind spot and detect early contraction of the peripheral limit due to glaucoma damage. The maintenance therapy of chronic glaucoma also requires that the physician understand the side effects of the drugs used in its treatment, from the well-known blurring effect of miotics to the less well-known production of subcapsular lenticular opacities from the use of the newer long-lasting drops (cholinesterase inhibitor).

In maintenance therapy the physician must also make sure that medication is taken or administered as prescribed. In the older age group it is wise before changing a therapeutic regimen because of apparent lack of therapeutic response, to ascertain that the patient or his medical attendant fully understand the importance of complying with the medication instructions as ordered.

Late Ocular Manifestations of Systemic Processes

Aging

The larger retinal blood vessels in the vicinity of the optic disks are true arteries and veins, being lined by a membrane called the intima, which is in contact with the blood column. All through life there is diffuse deposition of fibroelastic tissue in the vessel wall. There is progressively more fibrous than elastic tissue deposited resulting in relaxation of the vessel wall with widening and lengthening, accounting for the ophthalmoscopic appearance of widened light reflex and tortuosity, respectively. We also see multiple, small, rather round, yellowish bodies, especially between the disk and macula; these are subretinal colloid and hyalin excrescences, called drusen, on the innermost layer of the choroid and are of little functional significance unless heaped up in the macular region to interfere with central vision.

Atherosclerosis

Here, instead of or in addition to the diffuse subintimal thickening, nodular clogging deposits form on the intima, impeding blood flow, and resulting in occlusions such as we see in the blood vessels supplying the heart or the brain, including the carotid circulation which may produce unilateral blurring of vision (amaurosis fugax) and the vestibular-basilar system which may produce bilateral blurring of vision (visual claudication).

Hypertension

Hypertension may be superimposed on or hasten aging and atherosclerotic changes in the retinal veins and arteries, but the fundamental process is one involving the smaller arterioles.

Thus, hypertensive vascular disease of the retinal vessels is fundamentally one of arteriolar sclerosis, from the first stage of arteriolar narrowing through the second stage of nicking at the crossing of an arteriole and vein. The third stage is a retinopathy, when the arteriolar changes have resulted in retinal hemorrhages and exudates. The fourth stage is a neuroretinopathy with edema of the disc added to the vascular and retinal changes. The onset of the remonstrable changes in the retinal picture varies greatly from patient to patient, being accelerated in high diastolic and untreated cases. Headache, dizziness, and blurring vision, in the presence of positive ophthalmoscopic signs, are danger signals of impending stroke.

Diabetic Retinopathy

This is generally first manifested several years after the onset of diabetes by the appearance of microaneurysms, resembling and formerly called round hemorrhages. These are best seen in red-free light using the green filter on the ophthalmoscope. Later, hemorrhages and new blood vessel formations occur on the surface of the retina extending into the vitreous. These hemorrhages and the proliferative processes (retinitis proliferans) are the villains in the destruction of vision. Along with the retinopathy there may be a nephropathy with accentuated arteriosclerotic and hypertensive vascular changes in the fundus, and a neuropathy which may produce deviation of the eye by involvement of the extraocular muscles. These changes may occur in the presence of what appears to be adequate medical and dietary control of the disease, and indeed may occur later in life under these conditions.

Discussion

The foregoing material has been presented to acquaint the reader with the common signs and symptoms of the more-frequent eye conditions encountered in the aging population. In this way, the reader will be better informed as to the natural progress of the disease and when to call for assistance. This assumes that a base line has been established, and no one should undertake the maintenance of an elderly person without a documented evaluation of his ocular status. This report should include visual acuity for distance and near in the widely accepted Snellen and Jaeger notations, respectively; spectacle prescription with corrected visual acuity; visual-field charts with clearly outlined defects; the intraocular pressure as determined by the widely used Schiøtz instrument; and positive findings on external and internal examinations of the eyes with definitive instructions on medications, other treatment, and danger signs. Community programs to detect and watch vulnerable persons will serve a preventive function, but there is no substitute for base line data as an individual enters his senior years and possible confinement or disablement may restrict his access to medical resources.

The senior citizen is not stereotyped; his individual needs must be assessed. His visual acuity may be impaired but may be adequate for his circumscribed activities. On the other hand, optical aids may be indicated. These include different types of conventional spectacles, contact lenses in highly motivated aphakic cases, and magnifying devices. Many patients reach a point of stability in regard to spectacles, the accommodative and lenticular changes having attained a state of balance. Thereafter, decreasing acuity may be correlated with pathological processes not helped by conventional glasses. Others may experience the need for frequent changes of spectacles, for example, patients with maturing cataracts, chronic glaucoma, diabetes, or hypertension under treatment with certain drugs.

As mentioned previously in connection with postoperative cataract cases, contact lenses may be useful but should be reserved for highly motivated cases capable of handling them. The same applies to magnifying devices. The simplest and often the most useful is the simple magnifier, which may be hand-held or stand-mounted. It is important to remember that adequate illumination is essential, and that in general, the greater the power, the more restricted the field and the shorter the focal distance. For example, a 10x magnifier must be held one inch from the inspected material. If such a lens is mounted in a spectacle frame, this necessitates holding the subject matter at nose length. Such lenses corrected for aberrations are available in lightweight, shatterproof plastic. Prismatic loops for binocular use are also available, giving a magnification of approximately 2.25x at ten inches to 3.5x at four inches.

Spectacle magnifiers employing compact telescopic units mounted on spectacle lenses could give 1.7x to 3.0x magnifications from four feet to infinity. The patient looks through his ordinary spectacle lens but brings the telescopic unit into operation by slight elevation of the head. Reading caps are available to fit over the telescopic unit for near vision at convenient working distances for sewing, typing, drawing, and other activities. These devices require a residual visual acuity of at least 20/100 to 20/200.

These devices are merely gadgets without orientation for their use. The patient will be initially intrigued but will not persist in using them unless he understands both their limitations and advantages. Limitations imposed by light requirements, restricted range and field, compensatory body movements, and the necessary readjustments of spatial orientation and hand-eye coordination are not easy to overcome once the initial thrill of seeing more has passed. Vision is improved but circumscribed.

Various types of projection apparatus can enlarge images for easy viewing. A good example is the attachment older people have for the television screen. It is unfortunate, however, that with the growing geriatric population so little attention has been directed to human engineering. Even literature designed for senior citizens is often printed in Jaeger one- or two-sized type which requires maximum presbyopic correction under the best of circumstances but could be produced in Jaeger three- to five-sized type which is all many geriatric patients can read, and easier reading would also result in better comprehension, the latter also constituting a problem in some older people.

Summary

Optimal visual acuity in older people requires maximum glare-proof illumination and the best possible refraction and glasses. A large number of geriatric patients have adequate vision for their needs. Conservation and the best possible use of this vision is more important than imposing procedures which may be risky and prove to be a futile odyssey in the search for perfection.

Personnel involved in keeping older people at a functioning level should understand the common eye conditions which affect these people and be prepared to interpret, counsel, and reassure them, or to summon medical assistance when the indications arise. Eye specialists may not be readily available. General physicians can do an adequate examination with simple instruments and be prepared to take holding action until the services of an ophthalmic surgeon can be obtained.

A carefully prepared report of eye examination with recommendations should be in the hands of the responsible person in maintenance. This base line data is a must, not only in conservation of vision but in coping with problems as they arise. A standardized ocular profile can well be a community undertaking along with proper design for lighting and other equipment and a greater concern for older people in the preparation of reading and instructional material.

HEARING LOSS

The normal human ear is capable of discerning a wide range of pitch, but for hearing speech in everyday communicative needs, the band of frequencies corresponding to the three octaves above middle C on the piano keyboard, called the speech range, is the all-important one. The ear is also responsive to signals from the faintness of a pin dropping to the uncomfortable loudness of a pneumatic hammer. Accordingly, hearing loss at any frequency is expressed in a system of exponents called decibels. For example, a sixty-decibel (or sixbel) loss at one thousand cycles per second in the middle of the speech range simply means that it takes ten to the sixth power or one million times the loudness to attain threshold at that frequency, as compared to normal.

Types of Hearing Loss

Loss of Air Conduction

Air conduction loss is due to impedance of sound waves in the external canal or middle ear. Examples are middle ear disease and otosclerosis. In the latter, the impedance is generally at the oval window between the middle ear and the inner ear, where the air waves become fluid waves. The sensory nerve cells are stimulated by the fluid motion's sending impulses along the nerve of hearing for decoding in the brain into meaningful information. This type of hearing loss generally occurs earlier in life, so that if unsuccessfully treated either medically or surgically at that time, will persist into old age, when it may be present in advanced form. Amplification, however, will overcome the impedance giving intelligible hearing with a hearing aid. Persistent middle ear disease will require continuing otological care. Hopefully, however, the patient will have entered later life without a life-endangering chronic infection. There are simple causes of impedance, however, such as a wax plug in the external canal which can be removed easily.

Loss of Bone Conduction

Bone Conduction loss involves the perceptive apparatus and is appropriately called sensorineural, since either the sensory cells in the inner ear or the nerve of hearing are involved. Examples are damage due to noise and toxins.

Meniere's syndrome afflicts the inner ear, but an acoustic tumor involves the nerve of hearing. Both produce the perceptive type of loss and dizziness but may be differentiated by special tests. Perceptive hearing loss will be described further under age-related hearing loss.

Mixed Hearing Loss

Mixed Hearing Loss is a combination of both the conductive and sensorineural types and is not uncommon, for example, as a result of healed infection in earlier life and the high-tone loss which comes with aging.

Age-Related Hearing Loss

Age-related hearing loss is called presbycusis and consists of progressive loss for high tones with successive decade of life but often becomes stable in the seventh decade. As long as the loss is confined to high tones outside the speech range, adequate communicative ability is retained. If the speech range is invaded, a hearing aid may be necessary, but intelligibility of speech-hearing is often impaired, sometimes disproportionately with the same hearing loss in younger people.

Compensating for Hearing Loss

Hearing Aids

Hearing aids come in many makes, sizes, and forms, including body-worn, ear-level, and eyeglass types. The general indication is hearing loss below social adequacy in both ears. Application is usually made to the better ear for best amplification results. If one ear is at the borderline of social adequacy, the fitting may be made to the poorer ear if localization of sound is important. Application to both ears may be made for the same reason, namely, binaural localization. In general, however, the simplest and most economical application is best for older people, and only if indicated for the needs of the individual. As in the case of optical aids, the hearing instrument may become a nuisance and be abandoned unless the patient understands the limitations as well as the advantages of amplified sound, is motivated to listen attentively, and can manage its use.

Auditory Training

Auditory training is concerned with counselling in attentive listening and the proper use of a hearing aid. It is particularly important in a sensorineural type of hearing loss in which intelligibility of speech hearing is a major problem.

Speech Reading

Speech reading, also called lip reading, sometimes comes naturally in the patient's effort to improve his communicative ability. An instructional program, however, is preferable whenever available. Such a program teaches not only the interpretation of lip movements and facial expressions and gestures but also the integration of environmental clues in assessing the communicative situation. It is a valuable adjunct to a hearing aid and auditory training.

Discussion

The general principles applicable to maintenance of visual function apply here and will be briefly recapitulated. The responsible person or persons must understand what he is dealing with and what to expect. To this end, he should not assume the responsibility without a base-line medical report of deficits and recommendations on which to base his judgment, predicated on the actual needs of the patient for communicative adequacy and not on a quest for restoration to normalcy once possessed or even imagined. In this connection the therapist must be prepared to resist unrealistic persuasion which may prove to be both disappointing and risky. On the other hand, he must be ready to listen with empathy and to counsel, interpret, and convince authoritatively.

Summary

The maintenance of function in the geriatric patient should be considered in the framework of the total individual, including the special senses which provide him with information about his personal and physical environment and enable him to function appropriately.

Chapter XI

PUBLIC HEALTH MEASURES TO MAINTAIN GERIATRIC PATIENTS IN THE COMMUNITY

HARRY T. PHILLIPS

WHILE there are many definitions of public health (1), a broad one will be used in which the total community health aspects of the care of the aged are discussed. The term *public health measures* comprises organized community action taken by both tax-supported and voluntary agencies for the health care of the aged. Such action may be taken at national, state, or local levels. Many health agencies provide services which are available to any age group, yet it is known that they serve mainly the older citizen. Examples which readily come to mind are general hospitals, nursing homes, and a wide variety of clinics and chronic disease services.

Public health activities have traditionally emphasized preventive services as well as therapeutic or supportive services. Consequently, reference will be made to all forms of organized community action which provide health care, both to the potential patient and to the person who is already ill.

Although one distinguishes between official and voluntary agencies by the fact that the former is supported by tax money and the latter by contributions from private sources, voluntary bodies are becoming more dependent upon subsidies from tax sources. Conversely, official agencies often look to voluntary agencies for citizen participation, advice, and community support. Indeed, there is a steadily growing partnership between official and voluntary agencies, one of the characteristics of public health in the United States.

In addition to those arms of the Federal Government which have a direct responsibility for protecting the health of the nation, there are a number of offices and branches of the

Government which have an indirect bearing and influence on health programs. Most of these are located organizationally in the Department of Health, Education, and Welfare (2).

DEPARTMENT OF
HEALTH, EDUCATION, AND WELFARE*

This department is responsible for the main thrust of the Federal Government toward the improvement of health for all citizens but with major responsibility for the underprivileged and the especially vulnerable. The main operating agencies of the department are as follows, but only those offices which have programs identified with the health needs of the aged will be considered:

1. Public Health Service (which includes the National Institutes of Health, the Bureau of Medical Services, and the Bureau of State services).
2. Office of Education.
3. Vocational Rehabilitation Administration.
4. St. Elizabeth's Hospital.
5. Food and Drug Administration.
6. Social Security Administration (which includes the Division of Disability Operations which administers the Medical program).
7. Welfare Administration (which includes the Office of Aging and the Bureau of Family Services).

---

*At the time of printing of this book, the Department of Health, Education and Welfare and some of its component agencies were undergoing major organizational changes. In January, 1967, the United States Public Health Service was reorganized into five main operating bureaus: (1) Bureau of Health Services (which includes the Divisions of Community Health Services, Hospitals and Medical Facilities and Medical Care Administration); (2) Bureau of Disease Prevention and Environmental Control (which includes the National Center for Chronic Disease Control); (3) Bureau of Health Manpower; (4) National Institutes of Health; and (5) National Institute of Mental Health. The functions of the Gerontology Branch have been taken over by the Bureau of Health Services. Essentially, the changes have resulted in increased emphasis on solving the problem of the health manpower shortage, greater autonomy for the National Institute of Mental Health, and minor redistribution of functions of the old Bureaus of State Services and Medical Services. Further reorganization of the Department is likely to occur.

The department maintains regional offices with directors to provide coordination, evaluation, and general administrative supervision of agency programs. These seven offices are a major source of guidance and assistance to those seeking Federal aid for community health services. They are located in Boston, Massachusetts; New York, New York; Charlottesville, Virginia; Atlanta, Georgia; Chicago, Illinois; Kansas City, Missouri; Dallas, Texas; Denver, Colorado; and San Francisco, California.

United States Public Health Service

The United States Public Health Service began as an office in the Department of the Treasury in 1798. Through this office, weekly contributions were collected from the crews of ships in order to pay for hospitalization when sailors were away from home. This was, in effect, what today would be called a prepayment medical care plan.

Since that time the Public Health Service has grown into an agency which spends over two billion dollars a year. The three major operating Bureaus of the Service are the National Institutes of Health, the Bureau of Medical Service, and the Bureau of State Services.

National Institutes of Health

The Institutes comprises the main research wing of the service and is composed of several institutes, each concerned with a segment of medical science. Research is conducted intramurally (using its own staff and facilities) or is promoted and supported by the Institutes but carried out extramurally. These studies are conducted or administered by the National Cancer Institute, National Heart Institute, National Institute of Allergy and Infectious Diseases, National Institute of Arthritis and Metabolic Diseases, National Institute of Dental Research, National Institute of Mental Health, National Institute of Neurological Diseases and Blindness, Division of General Medical Sciences, and the Institute of Child Health and Development. Much of the research carried out by and through the National Institutes of Health is of direct importance to the maintenance of health of geriatric patients. Through these research funds, the staffs and facilities of medical schools throughout the country have been greatly strengthened and standards raised for patient care and teaching as well as for research. Some of the newer Federal health programs will probably help strengthen the ability of teaching hospitals to apply knowledge gained through research and thus increase the stress on patient care.

Bureau of Medical Services

This bureau is the medical arm of the Public Health Service and is primarily concerned with developing and directing certain medical care and health service programs. Direct care is provided for eligible beneficiaries to assist them at Public Health Service hospitals, outpatient clinics, and offices. Beneficiaries are mainly seamen, Coast Guardsmen, and other uniformed personnel as well as dependents of uniformed services personnel. Therapeutic and preventive health services are provided also for Indians through hospitals and health centers.

Bureau of State Services

This bureau is the principal operating bureau of the service for Federal-state and interstate programs. Its activities are promoted through two sections: the Environmental Health Section (concerned primarily with preventive services and includes Divisions of Aid Pollution, Environmental Engineering, Occupational Health, and Radiological Health) and the Community Health Section (concerned primarily with the care of patients at the community level).

Three Divisions of this bureau—Chronic Disease, Medical Care Administration, and Hospital and Medical Facilities—assist the states and localities in a variety of ways to improved health care of the aged (3). They promote the application of newer knowledge acquired through medical research or administrative demonstrations and provide assistance through standard setting, consultation, training, assignment of technical personnel, informational services, and the administration of grants-in-aid. The bureau's branches also conduct research and surveys and provide emergency aid to states.

DIVISION OF CHRONIC DISEASE

This division, which includes the Gerontology Branch, conducts a series of programs in specific categories of disease. For example, the Cancer Control Branch aims to lessen the gap between the discovery of new knowledge and its application at the community level. Tests and equipment for cancer detection are developed, and physicians' attitudes and practices concerning cancer are studied. Similarly, research activities, studies, and projects are supported in their respective fields by the Arthritis and Diabetes Branch, the Kidney Disease Program, the Heart Disease Control Branch, Neurological and Sensory Disease Branch, and the Chronic Respiratory Disease Branch.

In the Office of Preventive Services, studies and demonstrations are promoted for testing the effectiveness of early detection of disease. This office also supports the development of screening programs in which patients can be rapidly and economically tested for early-stage undiagnosed diseases. Screening programs do not aim to make definitive diagnoses but only to separate those persons who are more likely to have diabetes, heart disease, glaucoma, cancer, and other conditions and who require further diagnostic tests before a definitive diagnosis can be established.

The Gerontology Branch was added to the Division of Chronic Diseases in 1963. Services, research, training, and public and professional education are promoted. Its attention is directed to persons over forty-five years of age, and the importance of community self appraisal and the development of new patterns for providing community services is stressed. The branch promotes adult health conferences or periodic health appraisal, health education and counselling programs, screening programs for early disease detection, information and referral services, and the training and assignment of personnel. Such personnel assist in developing comprehensive programs and services in health departments, community hospitals, senior citizen centers, and housing projects.

The branch supports a number of research projects in the field of gerontology and studies of the patterns of utilization of services to the aged in various settings. Clinical psychologists who provide a course of training in dealing with aged patients as well as social science research in gerontology are also supported. Priority is given to professional education and training in applied gerontology, and to this end the branch works with universities; medical schools; schools of public health, nursing and social work; as well as official and voluntary agencies and professional societies. Continuing education programs in gerontology are being planned and promoted for all these key groups.

DIVISION OF MEDICAL CARE ADMINISTRATION

The Gerontology Branch acts as a focal point in the Bureau of State Services for all programs relating to the aging and aged. Liaisons are maintained with other Federal departments as well as with state agencies and voluntary and professional organizations concerned with the aged.

The Division of Medical Care Administration was established in August 1965, in order to assist the Social Security Administration in the implementation of Medicare, the health insurance for the aged program. This division has responsibility for medical care administration activities in general as well as specific responsibility for the professional health aspects of the new legislation. Professional standards for the program are set; training, evaluation, studies, and the development of utilization review plans are promoted; and relationships with the National Medical Review Committee—an advisory body assisting the Federal Government in the planning and implementation of the Medicare legislation—are established.

This division also provides consultation and technical assistance to other related programs in the Department of Health, Education, and Welfare and to other agencies concerned with the health insurance program. The division has responsibility for health economics and accordingly promotes and supports studies of the needs for services and their utilization.

The Nursing Home and Related Facilities Branch and the Home Health Services Branch of the division have corresponding responsibilities in their respective fields of the health insurance for the aged program. They are concerned with post-hospital or extended care in the nursing home or home setting and provide guide lines to assist in the training of personnel and services.

DIVISION OF HOSPITAL AND MEDICAL FACILITIES

This division was established through the Hospital Survey and Construction Act (Hill-Burton) in 1946. Through this program, large amounts of Federal monies have been provided to match state and local funds for the planning and construction of hospitals, health centers, rehabilitation centers, and nursing homes. Since the enactment of the program, the division has provided assistance for the construction of 54,000 long-term care beds in chronic disease and nursing home facilities. Through this program, too, funds are made available for administration, research, and demonstration in the provision of hospital facilities. The Hill-Burton funds also support training projects.

Other Divisions of Community Health Services

The Division of Dental Public Health and Resources provides consultation and technical assistance to state and local health agencies for the purpose of promoting dental programs at the community level. Research and demonstration projects are also supported. Particular interest is placed on the dental needs of older citizens. In a variety of projects, the dental needs of older people are being assessed, the feasibility of providing dental services in various settings is being investigated, and portable dental equipment is being developed. The division also promotes and supports training programs for dental students and practitioners.

The Division of Nursing aims to improve the understanding and skills of nurses working with geriatric patients as well as stimulate the development of services for home-bound patients. It participates demonstration projects for the establishment of homemaker services and community nursing services and the extension of public health nursing to areas not formerly served. It also supports studies concerned with the provision of community psychiatric nursing and training of nurses in geriatric care.

COMMUNITY HEALTH SERVICES AND FACILITIES ACT (1961)

This act added greatly to the impetus of the various programs of the Bureau of State Services in promoting or supporting out-of-hospital services for the chronically ill and aged (4). Among its many provisions are funds for *formula grants* and *project grants.*

Formula grants are given to state health departments to assist them in developing state plans for promoting community health services for the chronically ill and aged. The size of the grant for each state was based on a formula derived from the population and percentage of people over sixty-five years of age in each state and the economic status of the state. In some states, these monies mainly supported a single type of service such as bedside nursing, homemaker programs, or home care programs based upon county, district, or local health departments. In other states, greater diversity of services provided by both official and voluntary agencies were partly or wholly supported by Federal Chronic Illness and Aging formula grants.

Project grants, on the other hand, are awarded on a competitive basis to public or nonprofit agencies in response to applications for support of projects to promote community health services for the chronically ill and aged. In the first four years of the program the Public Health Service has approved 234 community health service projects. These funds have been applied to a wide range of methods for strengthening the communities' ability to care for the geriatric or chronically ill patient. Training of personnel providing home care, homemaker, nursing, or other home health services; establishment of central referral and information centers; experimentation with new methods of organizing community services; and the development of screening programs and artificial kidney services are some examples. The following is an example of a project specifically related to the health care of older people which was supported through Federal funds granted to a local agency.

QUEENSBRIDGE HEALTH MAINTENANCE SERVICE FOR THE ELDERLY

This project involved five official and three nonofficial agencies working under the direction of the New York City Department of

210 Maintenance Therapy for the Geriatric Patient

Health. Situated in a large public housing project in Queens, it provided a comprehensive health, medical, counseling, and follow-up service for about one thousand older persons residing in the project. The services offered were 1) periodic physical examination, 2) diagnostic and therapeutic services, 3) counseling, 4) referral, 5) follow-up, 6) housekeeping, and 7) recreational programs. These services originated in the Health Maintenance Clinic located in the housing project, but liaison was maintained with local health and hospital home care programs. This program was planned as a three-year demonstration and continued after the demonstration was over in a modified form.

In a number of instances, the Public Health Service, instead of making a grant, developed a contract with a nonprofit organization to provide a service, promote a training program, or conduct research because the agency was well equipped or located for carrying out this service. Many of these contracts have been made with state or local health departments, medical schools, or universities and have become an effective method of providing Federal support for local programs. Enactment of the Community Health Services and Facilities Act was a turning point in Federal assistance to local health agencies. The result was a major move away from the categorical approach, in which efforts are directed against a particular disease or group of diseases such as cancer or heart disease, to a more comprehensive approach.

Other Federal Programs Affecting Community Health Services

In an attempt to break the symptom complex of poverty, low educational status, unemployment, and poor health, the Federal Government has promoted a number of new agencies and programs. Some of these exert a direct or indirect influence on health or health services. Examples are the efforts by the Office of Economic Opportunity which aim to "eliminate the paradox of poverty in the midst of plenty in this nation by opening to everyone the opportunity for education and training, the opportunity to work, and the opportunity to live in decency and dignity."

Many of the community action programs established through this Federal agency have important health components. One such program aims to train older citizens with low incomes to become home health aides who can be usefully employed under the Medicare program. Similarly, the Appalachian Regional Commission in an economically depressed area of the country supports projects for a variety of facilities and services, among which are the construction and operation of multicounty health centers.

Public Health Measures by Official State and Local Health Agencies

By law, the individual states have primary responsibility for safeguarding the well-being of their citizens. State health departments, in turn, bear the responsibility for attending to the health aspects of this governmental objective. Other departments, however, such as Public Welfare, generally provide funds for purchasing health services for the needy; the cost of these services are met partially by Federal funds.

The Association of State and Territorial Health Officers, an organization consisting of the health commissioners of the fifty states, in 1964 adopted a statement defining the role of the state health department in providing services related to medical care. This document gives the following, and considered appropriate, functions and activities of some state health departments:

1. Planning and coordination.
2. Collection, interpretation and dissemination of information.
3. Research and evaluation.
4. Consultation, resource development.
5. Development and maintenance of standards and provision of services.

Naturally, the degree to which the various states perform these functions varies greatly. Nearly all state health departments have responsibility for regulating hospitals, nursing homes, and other institutions for the care of the sick. In some states, responsibility for nursing home regulation is placed in their welfare departments, although the tendency is to shift this over to health departments—an indication that nursing homes are increasingly being regarded as medical care facilities rather than charitable institutions.

Nearly all states have responsibility for licensing doctors, nurses, and other health professionals. Generally, these powers are in the hands of special licensing boards which have close relationships with the health department. In some states, the health department, in addition to providing institutional care for tuberculous and mentally ill patients, has become more and more involved in giving direct care for the chronically ill and aged. With the development of the new programs outlined in the Social Security Amendments of 1965, the medical care component of the state health program is destined to expand rapidly. Although few states provide the whole range of services outlined above, there are some which are giving medical care services beyond this range.

As can be seen from the description of the role of the Federal Government in providing medical care services, state health departments depend to a considerable extent upon support and stimulation from the Federal level. One of the weaknesses of the formula grant program is that matching funds, which are generally required, may not always be forthcoming, especially in the poorer states. Consequently, many needed programs are not developed for lack of money which could have been obtained through formula grants. Another weakness of the formula grant mechanism is that in many instances the highest priorities of need in a particular state cannot be met, but lower priorities can.

A comprehensive Health Planning and Health Services Amendment Act was passed in 1966. It will require each state to implement programs to serve the state's health needs. The various health grants are consolidated at the state level. This should give the state health departments greater flexibility and opportunities for using Federal grants to meet their needs as they see fit. The danger, however, is that local political pressures might be more readily felt if more decisions can be made at the state level.

In some states, the health departments have for a long time given direct services to particular groups of patients, for instance, patients with tuberculosis or other communicable diseases and the mentally ill and indigent. Since the decline of tuberculosis and communicable disease as a public health problem, an increasing number of sanatoriums are being converted to chronic disease hospitals. Such hospitals, it should be noted, are also supported by charity or local governments such as county or city. These chronic disease hospitals may or may not be associated with facilities for housing the homeless and indigent aged members of the community.

It is also important to remember that the difference between a chronic disease hospital and a nursing home, or infirmary, is that in the former instance there is a medical staff plus facilities for the diagnostic and therapeutic services which are not available in the latter type of institution. Nevertheless, it is often difficult to distinguish between the various types of institutions which are supported by tax funds derived from the state, county, or city budget for the chronically ill.

In recent years there has been a trend toward more active treatment and rehabilitation of the patient in the chronic hospital. Consequently, there has been a far greater turnover of patients in these hospitals with attempts frequently successful in getting the patient back home or into his community in a nursing home or similar facility.

In addition to institutional medical care, state health departments are providing a number of other community services specially aimed at the aging section of the population. In a survey of ten states reported by Graber (5), the following health services were provided by state health departments or, in some instances, local health departments:

1. Adult health conferences or health maintenance clinics were initiated to provide periodic health appraisal, health education, counseling, and referral services.

2. Health education activities were directed at the public rather than the professional. Special attention was directed at screening; accident prevention; nutrition; home care services; periodic health appraisal; and programs against diabetes, cancer, heart disease, and mental disease.

3. Screening may be provided for a single disease such as tuberculosis, diabetes, cancer, glaucoma, and hypertension or it may be provided for multiple conditions in the

same group of people. In some states, mobile units covered the territory. Patients found to be positive from the screening test were generally referred to their private physicians for more definitive diagnosis and treatment as indicated.

4. Information and referral service was provided in a number of states. Either the state health department or the county health department provided a professional staff to get information and make referrals for older patients requiring a variety of services.

5. Preretirement counselling was offered in a number of states through such channels as adult education offered by city public schools, chapters of the AFL-CIO, universities, churches, and Veterans Administration.

6. "Meals on wheels" programs were provided in some states. Frequently, these programs involved hospitals, community councils, churches, and commercial establishments as well.

7. Homemaker services were being offered or were being supported by a number of state health departments. These services provided assistance to families trying to cope with the problem of maintaining older patients in the home setting.

8. Home care activities were reported by a number of state health departments. In several states these were conducted by county health departments where services were given by nurses, nutritionists, physical therapists, and health educators to patients in their own homes.

9. Coordinated home care was supported by one city health department at the time of the survey. (However, there are a growing number of such programs based on voluntary agencies, and with the advent of the Medicare program it is likely that many more such services will be developed).

Since counties and cities vary greatly in size and wealth, it is to be expected that there would be a wide range of services for the health care of the older citizen in a different county and local health departments. Consequently, the great metropolitan areas such as New York, Chicago, and Los Angeles offer many services which are provided by state health departments and indeed are often minimal in many of the smaller departments. In smaller jurisdictions, community services for the geriatric patient provided by the official agency are likely to be very limited outside of the town infirmary of public medical institution; most services are provided by charitable or voluntary agencies.

Social Security and Welfare Administrations and Health Services

The horror of economic depression in the 1930's spurred the development of a number of reforms. The Social Security Act of 1935 initiated a series of social and public health measures which profoundly affected the well-being of the nation and especially the aged. Among the provisions of this and ensuing legislation was the development of a system of insurance and aid programs which today are administered by the Social Security Administration and the Welfare Administration of the Department of Health, Education, and Welfare.

The Social Security Administration is responsible, among other programs, for the following:

1. Old-age survivors and disability insurance which aims to provide continuing income for individuals and their families as partial replacement of earnings lost through old age, disability, retirement, or death.

2. Health insurance program for the aged (Medicare) which aims to ensure basic health services for the elderly. This program is described in another chapter.

The Welfare Administration is responsible for administering the programs of the Federal Government pertaining to individuals and families in need, and for providing welfare assistance and services for the aging and other groups. These programs are primarily Federal-state in nature with the states receiving Federal grants-in-aid in return for operating in accordance with Federal standards. This branch of the department includes the following sections which are relevant:

1. The Office of the Aging provides stimulation, guidance, and assistance to states, communities, and national organizations in the development of aging programs and services. The office serves as the coordinator of all aging activities of the Department of Health, Education, and Welfare. Naturally, many of its programs have a direct or indirect bearing on health services for the aging.
2. The Bureau of Family Services administers grants to help states provide public assistance under the Social Security Act for old-age assistance and medical assistance for the aged; aid to the blind, to the permanently and totally disabled; and similar services.

In the Kerr-Mills program (medical assistance to the aged), the Federal Government matches state payments for medical care for the aged who are needy. A major deficiency in this legislation is that the individual states have to take the initiative and decide the limits of services to be paid for. Consequently, a small number of states have established liberal programs, a number have none, and the remainder provide limited benefits. In all instances there is a means test which often prevents the older patient from seeking care or causing him to delay in doing so.

This bureau also administers Title XIX (Medicaid) of the Social Security Amendments of 1965. This title aims at the extension and integration of the various existing programs for the needy and also opens the way to improving the quality and comprehensiveness of their medical services.

These programs are to be administered through agencies designated in each state for the purpose; in most instances, the state department of public welfare has been so named.

Vocational Rehabilitation Administration

This branch of the Department of Health, Education, and Welfare aims to promote the greater utilization of disabled persons in gainful and suitable employment. The administration cooperates with the states in providing services to the handicapped. Services provided include medical diagnosis and treatment; supplying necessary devices such as artificial limbs and hearing aids; counseling, training, and placement. Before a person is considered eligible, the state agency must see that he satisfies three conditions: 1) have a disability which substantially interferes with employment, 2) have a reasonable chance of becoming suitably employed, and 3) be of an employable age. Consequently, only a limited number of older patients are likely to benefit.

VOLUNTARY HEALTH AGENCIES

Although voluntary agencies are not peculiar to the United States, they are more prominent in this country than in any other. They are supported through private funds, foundations, and/or subscriptions. Although their relative financial importance is decreasing and their role changing, it is likely that there will always be a need for voluntarism in the field of health (6), since the special quality of their services to the community cannot be provided entirely by governmental departments.

Voluntary agencies are of several types:

1. Organizations established to prevent or combat a particular disease or group of diseases. Examples of this type of agency are the National Tuberculosis Association, the American Cancer Society, The National Society for the Prevention of Blindness, the American Heart Association, and the National Safety Council.

2. Agencies supported through large philanthropic foundations such as the Rockefeller Foundation, the Millbank Memorial Fund, and many others serving smaller areas of the country. These have broad and sometimes changing objectives.

3. Associations representing professional workers in the health field. Examples are the American Medical Association, the American Public Health Association, American Nurses' Association, the American Hospital Association, and the like.

Over the years these associations have done great service in providing opportunities for citizen participation, promoting political reforms, setting standards, supporting research and demonstrations, promoting training and educational activities, and in supplementing services provided by official and private health agencies.

Of special interest in this context at the national level is the recently formed Association for the Advancement of Retired Persons which, among other activities relating to the well-being of older people, provides hospital insurance to its members. Similarly, the closely related Association of Retired Teachers includes among its many activities the provision of a service which obtains drugs and hearing aids for its members at reduced rates. With the advent of Medicare, the hospital insurance program and other health benefits offered by these groups will be changed to complement and supplement the government-sponsored insurance.

The Blue Cross-Blue Shield plans are also of great significance in providing funds for the health care for the aged. Although the plans are organized at the state or regional level, the various units are affiliated under a national body and are characterized by a uniform philosophy. These nonprofit, prepayment health insurance programs pool the costs and risks of expensive medical care, and by including the elderly, who are high-risk participants, they have had to raise premiums to all. However, by providing special coverage to the aged, the Medicare program will relieve the insurance plans of much of this responsibility so that they can now provide for some of those portions of health care not covered by Medicare. To a limited extent these plans have controlled the quality of care by stipulating standards of facilities which could participate in their insurance programs.

COMMUNITY HOSPITALS

In the typical American community, the voluntary hospital provides a central point for the medical care services of its citizens. In recent years there has been an increase in the number of older people in the community. They have a greater liability to become ill and require prolonged hospitalization.

At the same time there has been a reduction in childhood illnesses and communicable disease. Consequently, the median age of patients in voluntary hospitals in the last few decades has increased greatly. It is no exaggeration to say that the voluntary hospital today is largely a geriatric institution.

Hospitals had their origin in the need to provide shelter for the indigent sick. With the explosion of scientific knowledge in the health field, the hospital became the workshop for the practicing physician. Now a new phase emerges: the hospital is beginning to become the community health service center. Individual physicians are becoming less and less independent and are becoming part of a large organization, the hospital, which in turn is becoming integrated into a regional and national plan (7). Part of this change in the hospital and doctor's role is due to the increase in complexity and cost of medical care. A large part of the reason is the intervention of third party payers such as public assistance programs. Blue Cross-Blue Shield, and the Federal Government social insurance plans. With these developments in medical care, it is inevitable that there will be a greater degree of organization of health services. Standardization is inevitable, since third-party payers will insist on receiving a certain quality of care before they are willing to pay.

This trend is not recent, since the American Medical Association many years ago played a significant role in improving standards of medical training and practice, and more recently, together with the American College of Surgeons, the American College of Physicians, and the American Hospital Association, was instrumental in establishing the Joint Commission on Accreditation of Hospitals. This commission has had a remarkable influence in raising the standards of hospital care nationally.

Certain beginning trends in the regional planning of hospital care are bound to grow in the near future. The Bingham Associates Fund, operating in Maine since 1936, is generally considered to be the first example of regionalization in this country (8). However, there has been little growth of this pattern until recent years when regional planning councils began to develop in certain areas of the country. The rationale for developing regional plans stems from the desire to avoid gaps and duplications as well as from the growing shortage of personnel with the skills necessary to provide the services required. Hospitals and their boards and professional staffs will have to surrender a part of their autonomy and desire for prestige. Community leaders will not tolerate several hospitals in one small community offering rarely needed treatments, such as open heart surgery or expensive radiation therapy, when one hospital could serve all the community's needs. The motive to limit the rapid rise in the cost of hospital care is also driving communities to plan services more economically.

In a growing number of communities, the hospitals, whether tax-supported or voluntary, are beginning to show an interest in organized home care programs and are making better provisions for ambulatory services for patients who do not need to be admitted. No doubt the provisions of the Medicare plan will stimulate the growth of such out-of-hospital programs which will provide alternatives which are less expensive and may be socially and psychologically more desirable than institutional care.

Across the country there is evidence of experimentation with the organization of health services at the community level, often with the hospital as the center of a service. Increasingly, the community hospital, especially in the larger cities, is providing personal health care for individuals and families through its outpatient and emergency services. This applies especially to physician services required at night and over weekends.

NURSING HOMES AND RELATED FACILITIES

Since the development of Federal subsidies for old-age assistance and medical assistance to the aged, nursing home beds have increased in numbers very markedly. A nursing home is considered to be a facility established primarily for the provision of skilled nursing services for patients with chronic disease.

Some idea of the size and nature of the population cared for in such institutions is provided by the National Center for

Health Statistics. In 1965 an estimated 582,000 people were residents or patients in seventeen-thousand establishments which provide nursing or personal care primarily to the aging and chronically ill. Eighty-six per cent of this number are over sixty-five years of age. The population represents 5.2 per thousand residents in the country. The ratio of female to male residents is two to one, a reflection partly of the larger number of women in the older age brackets. Almost 20 per cent of residents were bedridden, and almost all the rest were confined to bed part of the time.

The national trend is for the total number of beds as well as for the average number of beds per home to increase. In most states the proportion of patients on public assistance in nursing homes is 70 per cent or more. Obviously, many patients are in such homes for social rather than medical reasons, since a large proportion of them are socially isolated as well as needy.

The great majority of nursing homes are privately owned and maintained for profit. In nearly all states the department of public health has responsibility for regulating homes and maintaining standards. Although the department of public health is primarily responsible for these standards, it works with the departments of public welfare, mental health and public safety, both at the state and local levels. In some states, nursing home owners and administrators have active organizations which have considerable potential for helping in the elevation of professional standards of care.

In the era before the enactment of the Social Security Act of 1935, maintenance of the needy, elderly, and infirm depended almost entirely on local community arrangements. The main sources of shelter and sustenance were religious and similarly charitable homes, the poor house, or public medical institution. While these sources have helped, they are becoming relatively less important.

In some areas of the country, community voluntary hospitals are developing long-term care facilities connected with the main institution. This arrangement has obvious advantages in that it may become possible to render better medical care to the patients. Under the Medicare legislation, the Federal Government reimburses agencies for reasonable costs without the ceilings which have in the past discouraged voluntary hospitals from giving long-term care and kept costs and, consequently, standards at a low level. This may result in the voluntary hospital's becoming more willing to accept responsibility for long-term care.

HOME HEALTH SERVICES

Traditionally, the home was the "proper" place for people to be cared for if they became ill. As indicated above, hospitals were established for those patients whose homes were inadequate for providing this care. For those who could afford it, the family physician visited and treated the patient in his home, and this arrangement was nearly always made on a personal basis between patient and doctor. Probably the earliest organized service to provide medical care at home was the Boston Dispensary program, established in 1796. The aims of the program were to save the sick from the pain of separation from their families, to lessen the expense of caring for the indigent sick, and to comfort the sick without humiliating them (10).

Since that time, physicians' home visits have become increasingly uncommon—for private patients as well as for others. Patients are much more frequently seen in doctors' offices, clinics, or in hospitals. However, the provisions of the Medicare legislation may have the effect of stimulating the development and greater use of health services in the home.

PUBLIC HEALTH NURSING

In addition to bedside nursing care, public health nurses render a number of health services such as the supervision of school health, maternal and child health, and participation in communicable-disease control programs. They are the most numerous professional group in public health and provide the main contact between health departments and other public health agencies and the public. In 1964 there were nearly 35,000 full-time professional nurses employed in public health work—a ratio of one nurse per 5,586 population (11). If subprofessional and part-time nurses were included, the number would be substantially increased.

Visiting nurses (or district nurses as they are sometimes called) were first employed by voluntary agencies; later, health departments began to use nurses for the wider range of functions now seen. Bedside nursing in the home, however, can be performed by nurses in both types of agencies. In some instances the nurse provides generalized services; that is, she combines various functions so that she may be rendering bedside care as well as child health supervision or communicable-disease control to the same families. Generally the visiting nurse will make only one visit to a patient without a physician's instructions. Nursing agency rules require nurses to visit thereafter only if a physician has seen the case and given orders for the nurse to follow.

A decrease in the utilization of visiting nurse services (12) in recent years has been evidenced. This is surprising, since there has been a general increase not only in population but also in the number of older persons in the community and a consequent need for chronic disease nursing. As mentioned above, it seems likely that many patients who could be cared for in their homes have been institutionalized. The designers of the Medicare legislation, by including home health services in the program, have taken an important step to promote care of the elderly in the familiar social and physical setting.

Public health nurses in agencies providing bedside care give far more than skilled nursing to the sick patient: They supervise family members or auxiliary personnel in giving nursing care; interpret the physician's findings and advice to the patient and family; assist in the patient's rehabilitation; prevent complications such as bedsores; advise the family on nutritional, financial, and emotional problems arising out of the care of the patient; or if they feel that the difficulties are beyond their capacity, know how to refer the family to community resources such as family or social agencies who can help; and assist the family and the patient in accepting referrals to the hospital, nursing home, or welfare department when these are necessary. Many public health nursing agencies provide their staff nurses with consultants in physical therapy, nutritional care, social service, and other professional consultation. These may be available within the agency itself or purchasable within the community.

In recent years, family service agencies and visiting nurse agencies have been promoting the use of homemakers or home health aides to help in the care of the elderly in their own homes. Whereas the homemaker has the broad function of maintaining the household, the main purpose of the home health aide is to give personal care under the supervision of a professional nurse who in turn is acting under medical direction. To a considerable extent, and with training, homemakers and home health aides are interchangeable. In 1963, the latest available report (13), there were 303 homemaker agencies in the United States, employing 3,906 homemakers who served 9,547 families. The last figure represented an increase of nearly 80 per cent over the number of families served in 1961. The rapid expansion of such services will certainly be accelerated by the Medicare program.

In a small number of communities, food services have been organized which provide "meals on wheels" to patients who are confined to their homes and have difficulty preparing satisfactory meals for themselves. Such services are still relatively undeveloped nationally.

COORDINATED HOME CARE PROGRAMS

A wide range of professional services exists for providing care in the home. Since 1947 there has been a steady pressure to develop mechanisms whereby the efforts of the various workers— physicians, nurses, social workers, nutritionists, physical therapists, and others—can be coordinated in the care of specific patients. Whereas care of the sick in the home is traditional, coordinated home care programs are relatively new. Several definitions are available, but a commonly used one is the following: "A coordinated home care program is one that is centrally administered and that through coordinated planning, evaluation and follow-up procedures provides for physician-directed medical, nursing, social and related services to selected patients at home" (14).

Programs of this nature are conducted generally by hospitals or by a variety of other community agencies—health departments, visiting nurse agencies, or medical schools. Admission to a program is in some, but not all, cases limited to patients on public assistance. The patient's medical condition should not require hospitalization, although he should need two or more kinds of professional care. Obviously, the home should be physically and socially suitable for such care. The growth of coordinated home care programs has been slow, but again it is anticipated that the provisions of the Medicare program will stimulate hospitals and other agencies to venture into new developments.

CONCLUSION

Taking an overview of community health services for the geriatric patient, the observer is struck by one finding—the great variability which exists in the quantity and the quality of the care which is available. The emphasis on individual initiative and on pluralism, together with reluctance to have the Federal Government, or for that matter any authority, dictate what to do sometimes results not only in impressive peaks in the standards of care but also in deep valleys in the standards of community services. Thus, rugged individualism can and does contribute both to the nation's strength and to its weakness in providing access to high-quality health care which older patients need. Much more can be done with our resources if and when community leaders agree to plan health and related services on an area-wide basis (15).

CASE HISTORY

The following case history is given to illustrate the collaboration which can develop between voluntary and official agencies in producing a community project for aiding in the health care of geriatric patients.

> In 1960 the community council of a medium-sized city, through its committee on aging, formed an Information Center for the Aging. The service was manned by personnel loaned by co-operating public and private agencies. Several voluntary agencies providing rehabilitation or recreation services began the collaborative plan with a group of five nursing homes and a VA hospital.

Because of the community interest in the well-being of the aged, a large private foundation awarded the committee a grant for studying the need for additional services for the aging and defining the policies necessary for creation of a useful pattern of working relationships between the various agencies involved in providing or paying for services to older people. The study revealed the need for a multiservice center for the people.

In 1960, representative citizens of the community formed an Age Center. In order to establish a demonstration which would implement recommendations of the study, the Center brought together voluntary and official agencies, health and welfare departments of the city, and the state health department. The latter assisted executives of the Center in drafting an application for a Community Health Services Grant by providing funds for an outside consultant. On several occasions, members of the staff of the Center and the Department of Public Health discussed drafts of the application with members of the regional office of the Department of Health, Education, and Welfare before final submission to the Public Health Service.

As a result of this activity, the Federal Government awarded a grant of over fifty thousand dollars a year for each of three years to demonstrate the use of the center for the aged for providing and coordinating a variety of health and social services needed by older people in apparently good health and by chronically ill persons.

Here in brief is an example of how public health measures stimulate community cooperation in providing activities which help to maintain the geriatric patient in the community.

REFERENCES

1. HANLON, J. J.: *Principles of Public Health Administration.* St. Louis, Mosby, 1964, pp. 23-24.
2. *United States Government Organization Manual.* Washington, D. C., Government Printing Office, 1965-66, pp. 344-372, 610.
3. GRABER, J. B.: A 1965 report of programs on aging. *Amer. J. Public Health,* 56:480-491, 1966.
4. *Bureau of State Services.* Report on planned activities for FY 1964, and anticipated activities for FY 1965 for the aging and aged.
5. GRABER, J. B.: *Presentation at the 17th Annual Meeting of the Gerontological Society.* Minneapolis, October 29, 1964.
6. HANLON: *op. cit.,* pp. 668-677.
7. ROSEN, G.: The impact of the hospital on the physician, the patient and the community. *Hosp. Admin.,* A:15-33, 1964.

8. ROEMER, M. I., and MORRIS, R. C.: Hospital regionalization in perspective. *Public Health Rep.*, 74:916-922, 1959.
9. WEINERMAN, E. R.: Changing patterns in medical care: their implications for ambulatory services. *Hospitals, 39*:67-74, 1965.
10. *150 Years of the Good Samaritan.* Boston, Boston Dispensary.
11. *Facts About Nursing.* New York, American Nurses' Association, 1965.
12. STEWART, W. H., and VAHEY, V. V.: Nursing services to the sick at home in selected communities. *Amer. J. Public Health, 54*:407-416, 1964.
13. *Directory of Homemaker Services, 1963.* Prepared by Medical Care Administration Branch, U. S. Public Health Service, Washington, D. C., 1963.
14. *Survey of Coordinated Home Care Programs.* Division of Chronic Diseases, U. S. Public Health Service, Washington, D. C., 1963.
15. *Areawide Planning of Facilities for Long-term Treatment and Care.* Report of the Joint Committee of the American Hospital Association-Public Health Service, U. S. Public Health Service, Washington, D. C., 1963.

Chapter XII

THE MEDICARE PROGRAM AND ITS SIGNIFICANCE FOR MAINTAINING THE GERIATRIC PATIENT

JAMES C. HUNT

T HE EIGHTY-NINTH Congress legislated the most comprehensive program for the elderly in our nation's history: the Health Insurance for the Aged Act, commonly known as Medicare. This program will be of primary significance in maintaining the geriatric patient. Its implementation and application will provide a primary economic thrust for improving and enlarging the spectrum of the sociomedical constellation and those services now available to the older American who suffers chronic ailments and illnesses.

The new Medicare legislation has been likened to a three-layer cake, the first two layers being the hospital insurance plan and the medical insurance plan of Title XVIII of the Social Security Act and the third layer being the Title XIX welfare provisions for medical care. Title XIX greatly expands the previous public assistance provisions of the Kerr-Mills legislation and establishes a standard of payment of reasonable costs for health and medical services furnished to public assistance recipients. This latter provision will ensure that hospitals and other health agencies will not be asked to subsidize the medical service they provide to persons receiving public assistance aid.

Title XIX increases the Federal funds available for state medical programs for indigent persons. The intent is to make health and medical services available to all needy persons, regardless of age. Low-income-family children under age twenty-

228

one can receive medical care under this program (if the state so elects) even though their parents are not receiving public assistance. The additional Federal funds made available under this program will ease the burden of expenditures which the states now have to bear because of public assistance programs. It is hoped that the states in turn will place more money into their medical program.

In order to be eligible for the funds under Title XIX, the states are required to combine all their medical assistance programs under one administrative entity and provide five minimum services: inpatient hospital care, outpatient hospital care, physician services, x-ray and laboratory services, and skilled nursing home services for adults only. They have to provide health and medical care to all indigent persons and not just the elderly as was required heretofore under the Kerr-Mills legislation. Title XIX will serve as a great incentive for having states expand and improve the quality and quantity of their present medical assistance programs. These Federal funds must be matched on a more modest scale than heretofore.

Medicare is a program devised to help pay the costs of medical services, not to provide the medical services per se. These services will still be furnished by physicians, hospitals, nursing homes, nurses, therapists, home health aides, and the trained workers in supportive disciplines. On this point Arthur E. Hess has stated.

> The health insurance program neither would provide services nor control the rendering of service. It would operate no hospitals, hire no physicians to practice medicine, and treat no patients. It is designed to pay the cost of services after they are rendered. The responsibility for and the control over the medical services furnished a beneficiary would continue to rest entirely with the physician and the institutional provider of services. The bill specifically prohibits the Federal Government from exercising supervision or control over the practice of medicine, the manner in which medical services are provided, and the administration and operation of medical facilities. Each provider of services would be free to decide whether or not to participate in the program, and an agreement to participate could be terminated if the provider so decides. A beneficiary would not be restricted in his choice of the institution

or medical practitioner. As under conventional hospital insurance and third-party prepayment programs, the physician determines for his patient the services that are medically necessary, and the health insurance program meets the cost or charges, as the case may be, for services that are covered.

The distinction between the payment of costs and providing medical services is important because some critics have stated that the Medicare program is going to engender bitterness. They claim that there are just not enough medical facilities and health personnel available to provide services for the number of people who will now be able to afford such services because of Medicare. If an inordinate patient influx should develop, and the present medical complex proves inadequate to deal with the situation, the fault should not be attributed to this great insurance effort but to those socioeconomic forces which have heretofore inhibited the necessary development of adequate facilities and personnel to care for all the people. Some critics also claim that because of an increased patient influx there is bound to be a decline in standards of medical care.

To achieve some conception of the present condition of medical manpower in the United States, note the following excerpt from the article "Crisis Now Near in Medical Care?" which appeared in the March 7, 1966 issue of the *U. S. News and World Report* (page 41): "Only now has a complete census of the U. S. medical personnel been undertaken. The last one was made in 1958. The present tally will be completed, it is hoped, in May, and Medicare begins in July."

Some preliminary figures and educated guesses are available, however, to point out what kinds of medical workers, besides nurses, are in dangerously short supply:

Anesthesiologists

"A lack of competent anesthesiologists is a serious bottleneck" according to Dr. E. M. Papper, Consultant to the National Institute of General Medical Science. He adds, "With scarcely enough anesthesiologists for routine surgery, complex operations like open-heart or brain surgery often require as many as three anesthesiologists. We have 8,500 specialists and we need 3,500 more. We only turn out three-hundred to five-hundred a year."

Radiologists

The American College of Radiologists reports that there are 9,600 doctors in the United States specializing in x-ray work. The need now is for twenty-thousand. Only five-hundred are being trained each year. The amount of x-ray diagnosis and treatment is mounting steadily. There were 100 million x-rays given in 1961 and 108 million in 1964. Medicare will probably vastly expand the demand.

Pathologists

"We have 5,600 clinical pathologists doing delicate and vital diagnostic work in the U. S. now, and we could use two-thousand more," says Oliver J. Neibel, Jr., of the College of American Pathologists. He points out that a complete physical checkup now calls for seventeen laboratory tests, whereas ten years ago only nine were called for. He adds, "we're relying on part-time helpers for assistants and technicians and running the risk of sloppier laboratory work."

Pharmacists

Dr. Bonnet of the AHA told a national conference on health-manpower needs on February 15, "Some 45 per cent of our hospitals do not have a pharmacist on their staff in spite of the fact that the number of full and part-time pharmacists in hospitals was six-thousand in 1962." He estimates that ten-thousand will be needed by 1975.

Technicians

Just as dangerous as the shortage of highly-trained professional men and women in the health fields is the shortage of technicians. This is the view of Dr. Harvey I. Scudder, Chief of the Health-Manpower Division of the Public Health Service. Dr. Scudder's guess is that "by 1970 the U. S. will need 172,000 skilled medical technologists to operate the new wave of modern scientific equipment now coming into hospitals. There are only 38,000 people in the country qualified to do this work today."

These general shortages affect medical care for people of all ages, Dr. Scudder points out.

In addition, he sees shortages which will hit old people particularly hard when they seek the benefits of Medicare. Chief among these lacks, Dr. Scudder says, is that of physical therapists. These practitioners, although not MD's, are as important as internists or surgeons in keeping older people active and useful to themselves and others.

"There are only twelve-thousand physical therapists in the U. S. There is need for twenty-thousand. By 1970, the need will be forty-thousand. The 1966 graduating class is about one-thousand. Critical as the shortages of medical manpower will be all along the line when Medicare gets going, many authorities see much worse to come."

These shortages were in existence before the inception of Medicare, and their resultant shortcomings should be in no way attributed to this great new program. Furthermore, medical standards which can be maintained only by failing to provide medical care to large numbers of Americans are certainly not desirable or enviable standards; one could almost term them inadequate standards. Besides, there can be no doubt that this great nation with its vast economic and human resources cannot help but win this war on ill health and disease now that this immense medical care offensive has been launched.

Arthur E. Hess stated, "The proposed hospital and health insurance program for the aged will not only provide relief to the pressures on public assistance funds but will provide significant relief to the premium rate structure of insuring organizations like Blue Cross that have been struggling to provide adequate health benefits to the high-risk, low-income groups that typically constitute the over-sixty-five population. The assumption by the new Medicare program of a large part of the fiscal task of insuring the elderly could stimulate private insurance and prepayment organizations to be more creative in improving voluntary health benefits protection, with particular attention to the 90 per cent of the population under age sixty-five, and also by providing new kinds of insurance protection supplementary to the Government program for those over sixty-five. A new kind of partnership is seen as likely to emerge in which Government and private agencies each would concentrate primarily on financing health for different segments of the population and would use administrative mechanisms in the voluntary sector to work toward the solution of common problems. Such a partnership will require greater public accountability as well as concentrated planning on the part of private organizations.

The challenge to planning organizations can be stated simply: The health insurance program can help put services within economic reach of older citizens, but further planning is required to make sure that voluntary as well as governmental programs for the expansion and rational use of manpower and facilities bring these services within practical reach. There are many communities from coast to coast which have the basic components to render effective and more comprehensive care to older citizens. With the expectation of new sources of financing—assured reimbursement for services to patients—what is lacking in facilities and organization must now be quickly brought into focus for community planning and community action.

It will take time and a dedicated effort on the part of all to work out satisfactory solutions to the program and administrative problems common to both public and private measures for preparing or otherwise financing medical services. While their problems may lend themselves to grass-root solutions, energetic leadership is required in the voluntary sector as well as in state and local government to assure planning and coordination of programs to the point at which financing and delivery of services to the individuals come together. By providing patient income for a comprehensive range of services, the proposed new program should encourage states, communities, hospitals, and the medical profession to plan for a more rational expansion and use of facilities and to offer the consumer appropriate and less costly alternatives. All shall have to work hard—and work shoulder to shoulder—to convert potential into reality.

It is felt that the program of health care for the aged—working through established organizations and health care institutions which will participate essentially as agents of the public in the administration of the program—can be made to work in ways which will enhance the quality as well as quantity of service and the variety of arrangements which is so characteristic of a free-enterprise society.

Many authorities believe that the critics are unduly apprehensive and that no unmanageable patient load is going to develop. Dr. Harold M. Granning, Chief of the Public Health Service's Hospital Division, "is not too alarmed about this prospect. Patients over sixty-five already make up about one quarter of the current hospital load. Under Medicare old people will gain, in addition to hospitalization, much more home and office care than they now receive, and they will also be eligible for largely cost-free care in nursing homes. There will be some strain where the occupancy rate of hospital beds is already near the limit but not to a critical degree elsewhere."

It is impossible to foretell what effect Medicare will have on hospital bed needs. However, because safegards are built into this program, it possibly may not result in any unnecessary burdensome overcrowding of hospital facilities. The necessity for physician certification of medical need for services, the deductible on hospitalization, the condition for hospital and extended care facility utilization review committees, and the coverage of alternatives to hospital care will lessen the impact on these facilities and provide controls to help prevent overcrowding.

The home health care provision will enable persons requiring a lesser degree of care to receive medical treatment and services at home for specified periods of time. The aged represent only 20 per cent of hospital bed users. In addition, full payment of bills by patients plus the funds available from the Hill-Burton program, the hospital modernization program, and other Government-related programs will enable hospitals and other facilities to expand existing structures or build new ones and train additional health personnel. With adequate funds made available there can be no doubt that the genius of the medical and hospital complex can more than adequately handle the situation.

Immediate access to proper medical evaluation and treatment should be available to every older American, not merely to those whose economic circumstances happen to be more fortunate than most. If, when Medicare becomes operational, the nation is faced with a shortage of medical manpower, paramedical personnel, and trained professional personnel in supportive disciplines, it is this deficiency which must be examined and remedied. Fortunately, the medical profession and the Government are studying and readying measures to remedy the situation if any shortage of facilities should develop. There can be little doubt that two of the biggest industries in the second half of the twentieth century are going to be the health and education fields, and there are no two disciplines which can have a more beneficial effect for all mankind.

While the quality and quantity of medical facilities and services have grown immeasurably over the years, the geographical distribution of these facilities and services is uneven. In many areas of the country there are far too few facilities and trained personnel. However, Medicare, by ensuring that the providers of medical services will be paid the reasonable costs of these services, provides a major incentive for the growth of such services. In addition, the Federal Government through the Hill-Burton Act and related programs provides funds for construction and implementation of hospitals, nursing homes, and other health facilities and services.

✓Medicare and the many other Government programs designed to aid the development of medical care make possible one of the greatest advances toward improved health and social progress. Economic barriers to properly needed medical care are removed. Now the elderly will be able to receive treatment when they need it and will not be deprived by financial want. They will be able to have their ailments propitiously treated in initial stages and not, as so often happened in the past, postpone treatment until the pain or discomfort became so unbearable that they could not stand it and were forced to seek treatment, only to discover that it was too late for any worthwhile remedial action.

It is impossible to estimate how many elderly persons consigned themselves to chronic invalidism or an earlier death by excessive postponement of medical treatment because they could not afford it. It is impossible to minimize the tremendous physiological and psychological damage wrought on elderly people because of failure to seek proper medical attention at the inception of an ailment because of economic deprivation.

In order to visualize the economic impact which illness has on elderly persons and why so many postpone visiting a physician, one has only to consider the marginal economic existence which a great many older Americans lead. William D. Bechill, the United States Commissioner of the Administration on Aging, in appearing before the Special Committee on Aging of the United States Senate on January 20, 1966, testified.

> One third of our older Americans live either in the homes of their children or in rented quarters. Many of them are one-room walkups, run-down hotels, old lodging houses or isolated farm houses. Rent for such accommodations often takes one third of their total income.
>
> Food expenditures for couples at the poverty level is about twenty-three cents a meal or seventy cents per person per day. Every meal—year in and year out—must be eaten at home. Under even a somewhat more liberal budget, one suit is budgeted for a man every three years, one pair of shoes a year, and a new necktie every two years. Women, on the basis of this budget, may have a suit every three years, a skirt every five years. The elderly on the poverty level, with plenty of time to read, can buy one newspaper per day, one paperback book and one magazine subscription per year. They can afford only two bus fares per person per week. They can purchase one television or radio set during the entire retirement period and spend not more than one dollar and twenty-two cents a year for repairs. One fourth of the elderly poor are without telephones.
>
> These are some of the personal dimensions of poverty among older Americans. The enactment of Medicare and the other important features of the Social Security Amendments of 1965 represent additional weapons to protect the financial and personal independence of retired people.

From this testimony the tragic impact of the skyrocketing costs of medical care to the aged can be readily visualized. Until now, illness and hospital costs were an unbudgetable item for most of the aged. Medicare now makes these expenses more budgetable, and for the first time almost all the elderly can now obtain care when they need and want it.

The Health Insurance for the Aged Act, which is commonly referred to as Medicare, provides two kinds of basic health insurance protection: hospital insurance, which is also termed Part A; and the supplementary medical insurance, termed Part B, which requires the three-dollar monthly premium.

Nearly every American sixty-five or over will be protected under the hospital insurance program beginning in July 1966. Hospitalization for up to ninety days in a "spell of illness" is provided for. A spell of illness begins on the first day an elderly person receives covered services in a hospital. It ends after the person has been out of a hospital or extended care facility for sixty consecutive days. The patient may be discharged and readmitted several times during a spell of illness, but a new spell of illness cannot begin until a patient has been out of a hospital or extended care facility for sixty consecutive days. The program pays for covered services during the first sixty days of care in a participating hospital, except for the first forty dollars. If the person is hospitalized for more than sixty days during a spell of illness, Medicare will pay all but ten dollars daily for covered services during an additional thirty days of care. There is a lifetime limitation of 180 days on payments for treatment in mental hospitals.

Medicare also provides for part payment of outpatient hospital diagnostic services. It will pay 80 per cent of the cost for diagnostic services an elderly person receives as an outpatient of a participating hospital during a twenty-day period, except for the first twenty dollars for each twenty-day period. This outpatient diagnostic service provision can lead to improved, enhanced service in hospital outpatient clinics. Outpatient treatment grows increasingly more important because of the diminishing number of general practitioners and the rising costs of hospitalization.

There is also a provision for part payment of post-hospital extended care. After a mandatory three-day stay in a participating hospital and providing that the patient is admitted within fourteen days from the date of hospital discharge, Medicare pays for twenty days' care in what is termed an extended care facility which is a sort of skilled nursing home. If a patient needs this care for more than twenty days during a spell of illness, the program will pay all but five dollars daily for an additional eighty days. The reason there is a mandatory requirement for a three-day stay in a hospital prior to admittance to the extended care facility is to ensure that the patient's medical condition and needs will have been medically gauged by the extensive facilities which are available only in hospitals. This will promote an adequate medical work-up and diagnosis to determine the proper nursing home therapeutic program to be planned for the patient's welfare. Medicare is a program designed to be therapeutic and not merely custodial in nature.

It is readily discernible that Medicare's post-hospital extended care provision does not provide for long-term nursing home care. The patient exhausts this benefit after one-hundred days during a single spell of illness. Of course if he experiences more than one spell of illness, he is then allocated up to one hundred days during each spell of illness. As has been pointed out before, the purpose of Medicare is not custodial care but therapeutic care. Another reason for the comparatively short period of post-hospital extended care benefits was recognition that skilled nursing homes are in short supply and that this limited period would contribute to a more rapid turnover and greater availability of nursing home beds for more people.

However, there can be no doubt that when this program becomes operational, if certain needs arise, the American people and Congress will ameliorate these needs by providing the necessary legislation. It must be remembered that Medicare is a program of limited benefits.

Medicare also has a post-hospital home health care services provision. The program will pay the costs for up to one hundred visits during the 365 days following a patient's discharge after a stay of three days or more in a hospital or extended care facility, if these services are furnished under a plan established and supervised by a physician. Covered under the home health services category are part-time or intermittent nursing care by or under the supervision of a registered nurse; physical, occupational, or speech therapy; medicosocial services under the direction of a physician; to the extent permitted in the regulations, part-time or intermittent services of a home health aide;

medical supplies (other than drugs and biologicals) and the use of medical appliances; and medical services of interns and residents-in-training under an approved teaching program of a hospital with which a home health agency may be affiliated.

The architects of the Medicare legislation hope to achieve in the area of home health services a program of post-hospital home care, supervised by a physician and under the control of an agency with established policies and set procedures. The home health care provisions, coupled with the extended care facilities measures, will help ease demands on hospital facilities, and patients requiring less intensive care will be able to receive it at less expense. Also the outpatient diagnostic services plan will enable patients to obtain diagnostic services without admission to a hospital.

There can be no doubt that there is a great shortage of the home health care facilities. However, the funds made available for payment of the reasonable costs of extended care and home health care services will provide a great economic incentive for the establishment and expansion of such services to meet these needs. In the future a great many hospitals will establish extended care facilities and operate home health care agencies. This program cannot help but make for a more closely knit complex of the present constellation of diverse medical services.

The hospital insurance program helps the patient pay his hospital bills, but it does not pay his bills for physicians' and surgeons' services. However, the elderly person can provide in advance for paying his doctors' and surgeons' bills and other medical bills too by enrolling in the voluntary supplementary medical insurance part of the Medicare bill. Entailed is the payment of a small monthly premium of three dollars by the enrollee with the Federal Government matching this amount.

The voluntary supplementary medical insurance program pays 80 per cent of the reasonable costs or charges for covered services, except for the first fifty dollars in a calendar year—the elderly individual has to pay this fifty-dollar deductible. This covers physicians' and surgeons' services, home health visits, and other medical and health services. No matter where the elderly person receives the physicians' and surgeons' services—at home, in the doctor's office, in a clinic, or in a hospital—he is covered under this part of the program.

Also the medical insurance plan entitles a beneficiary to one hundred home health visits under an approved plan each year with no need for prior hospitalization. This benefit is in addition to the one hundred visits provided under the hospital insurance program. Thus, an elderly person who has subscribed to pay the three-dollar premium for the supplementary medical insurance would be entitled to two hundred home health visits a year if he were hospitalized for at least three days—the one hundred visits provided under the hospital insurance program plus the one hundred visits provided for under the medical insurance part which requires no prior hospitalization.

Other medical and health services, regardless of where rendered, included under the medical insurance coverage are such things as diagnostic tests (x-rays and so on), laboratory services; x-ray or radium treatments; surgical dressings, splints, casts; certain ambulance services; braces, artificial legs, arms, and eyes; rental of medical equipment such as iron lungs; and many other medical items and services.

The above benefits afford all geriatric patients the most comprehensive program of medical services in our nation's history, and the financing of this program through Social Security taxes provides funds that were never before available to the health care field on such a large scale. The ramifications of Medicare are bound to have the most tremendous impact on the financing and organizing of medical care in the nation's history. Improved and more extensive utilization of all types of health care facilities are built into this program. Preventive maintenance therapy and progressive health care of the geriatric patient is now more feasible than ever before, thanks to the extended care and home health provisions.

The administration of this comprehensive program is bound to be a mammoth undertaking. This administration will involve Federal and state agencies, hospitals, nursing homes, and home health associations and private insurance companies.

Apropos of this aspect, Arthur E. Hess has stated,

Successful administration, then, will call for cooperation and leadership in their organizations of physicians, hospital boards and administrators, public welfare officials, voluntary agency personnel, third-party prepayment and insurance executives, and state and local health officers. The bill, in fact, recognizes the need for and provides financial support to planning activities at the community and state levels. In order to bring into perspective the impact of the new program and to provide appropriate coordination with those other programs, public and private, that have to do with the construction, expansion and better utilization of services and facilities, the Medicare program (through appropriate state and local agencies) may bear a fair share of the costs of certain planning activities.

In order to qualify for participation in this program, hospitals, extended care facilities, and home health agencies must meet certain specified conditions. Each of these providers of medical services is free to decide whether or not to participate in the Medicare program, and any agreement to participate can be terminated whenever the provider wishes.

Hospitals must be licensed by the state. In those states which do not require licensing, compliance with the state or local law governing the certification or approval procedures of hospitals will fulfill this licensing requirement. In addition, hospitals must comply with requirements relating to utilization review, adequate maintenance of clinical records, medical staff bylaws, and other specified conditions. The law authorizes the Federal Government to institute any further standards necessary to the health and safety of Medicare beneficiaries. These standards cannot be stricter than comparable requirements of the Joint Commission on Accreditation of Hospitals.

Those hospitals accredited by the Joint Commission on Accreditation of Hospitals will generally be conclusively presumed to meet all the conditions for participation. There is a definite requirement that a utilization review committee be established as a safeguard against unwarranted use of hospital facilities. This board would review periodically on a sample basis the admissions of Medicare beneficiaries, the need for the medical services provided, and the length of stay. The hospital can establish its own utilization review committee or it can join a community-based utilization committee sponsored by a local medical association in cooperation with other hospitals and other providers of medical services. This procedure will encourage the optimum use of hospitals and the services they afford.

There are also regulations governing the participation of the extended care facilities. An extended care facility can be a skilled nursing home, or it can be a distinct part of an institution such as a ward or wing of a hospital, or it can be a facility, one part of which is an old-age home. The extended care facility must provide around-the-clock nursing service for sick or disabled persons with at least one registered nurse employed full time. Every patient must be under the care of a physician, and a physician must be available to handle emergencies. Appropriate policies must be maintained governing the home's nursing care and services. There must be appropriate methods for handling and dispensing drugs. The extended care facility must maintain clinical records on all patients and have a utilization review plan. In addition, the law allows the Federal Government to prescribe further requirements necessary to protect the health and safety of Medicare beneficiaries.

The extended care facility must also have a written transfer agreement with a hospital or hospitals for the transfer of patients and the exchange of clinical records. A transfer agreement with any participating hospital would qualify the extended care facility to receive patients and provide post-hospital care to patients transferred from other hospitals with whom it did not have a transfer agreement. If the extended care facility had tried in good faith to arrange a transfer with nearby hospitals but was unsuccessful, the state agency assisting in the administration of the Medicare program may waive the requirement for a transfer agreement if the agency finds that the extended care facility's participation in the hospital insurance program is in the public interest and essential to assuring this type of care to the elderly people in the community. This regulation will assure the maintenance of good standards for the therapeutic care of patients.

The requirements for home health agency participation are intended to assure that the agency is a provider of health services. The home health agency must be primarily engaged in providing skilled nursing and other therapeutic services and have policies established by a professional group associated with the agency which includes at least one physician and one registered nurse to govern their services. It must be approved by the appropriate state agency, maintain clinical records on all patients, provide for supervision of its services by a physician or registered nurse, and meet other conditions of participation as the Secretary of the Department of Health, Education, and Welfare may find necessary in the interest of the health and safety of individuals who are furnished services by the agency.

This part of the program covers visiting nurse organizations and home health services provided by a hospital as well as agencies specifically established to provide a wide range of home health services. The home health agency must be publicly owned, or be a nonprofit organization exempt from Federal taxation, or be licensed and meet staffing requirements and other standards and conditions prescribed by regulation. An organization providing home care on a profit basis may qualify if it is licensed, where state law requires it, and if it meets specified standards.

The physician plays the key role in the Medicare program. Payment will be made only if a physician certifies to the necessity of the services rendered. It is the physician who decides upon an admission to a hospital, the method of treatment, and the length of stay. The physician will also have to certify that outpatient hospital diagnostic services were necessary in order to have such diagnostic studies paid for under Medicare.

Physician certification is also necessary to qualify for payments for extended care and home health facility treatments. Under the program the reasonable costs of services ordinarily provided to inpatients by hospitals will be paid for. The nursing services which hospitals ordinarily provide will be paid for, but private duty nursing is now covered. Hospital room and board in semiprivate (two to four beds) accommodations will be paid in full. If the patient's condition requires him to be isolated in a private room because he has a communicable disease, then the cost of the private room will be fully paid. However, if the patient has a private room merely for personal comfort, the program will pay the semiprivate rate, and the patient will have to make up the difference. Drugs, biologicals, supplies, appliances, and equipment ordinarily furnished to inpatients by the hospital are fully covered. Other diagnostic and therapeutic services ordinarily furnished by the hospital to its patients will be paid.

Services by medical and dental interns and residents-in-training if they are under a teaching program approved by the American Medical Association, American Osteopathic Association, or American Dental Association are covered. However, payments will not be made under the hospital insurance plan for medical or surgical services provided by physicians, and this exemption includes the services of radiologists, anesthesiologists, pathologists, and physiatrists; their services are covered under the medical insurance plan of Medicare.

Services and items generally provided by extended care facilities will be paid for by Medicare. These include room and board in semiprivate accommodations except when more expensive accommodations are medically necessary; nursing care by or under the supervision of a registered nurse; physical, occupational, or speech therapy; and medicosocial services. Payment can also be made for the medical services of interns and residents-in-training and other diagnostic and therapeutic services provided to inpatients of the extended care facility by a hospital with which it has a transfer agreement. Payment can also be made for occupational, physical, and speech therapy provided by entities other than the extended care facility, if provided under conditions which stipulate that payment for the therapy be made through the extended care facility. Items and services which are not covered in a hospital are not covered in an extended care facility.

The number of skilled nursing homes is limited, and far too many nursing homes are merely custodial in nature. This new health insurance program will constitute a tremendous stimulus to the construction and growth of new, skilled nursing homes and the conversion of many which are merely custodial in nature to the skilled category. Also, the financial support which this insurance program affords to the home health agency type of service will furnish an incentive to the growth of the number of these agencies to accommodate this important area of medical need.

The outpatient hospital diagnostic services provisions will lead to greater utilization of the important functions which outpatient clinics fulfill. Outpatient departments will screen out the aged who do not need hospitalization and can chart treatment or therapeutic courses for them. This method will preclude unnecessary hospitalization.

It can be readily seen that Medicare encompasses the full, broad spectrum of medical services; the provisions of this far-reaching compassionate law provide for payment of hospital, skilled nursing home, home health care, outpatient clinic, and private physician services to our aged population. A new era is dawning in the maintenance of geriatric patients. However, the Medicare program is only a beginning—a very good beginning—but much will remain to be done. Developing experiences with the program will evidence what must be achieved in order to see that the aged population receives complete medical services.

Now, fairly comprehensive, coordinated, and continuous health programs can be planned and developed for almost all the aged, and if any shortcomings develop they can be remedied by concerted action. Awesome financial barriers have been removed for the aged. All too often in the past, our aged, because of economic deprivation, hesitated to seek medical treatment until it was too late. Now they can seek treatment at a more propitious moment.

From the complex of medical services which will be put within economic reach by Medicare, maximum flexibility and adaptiveness of treatment can be planned, with the ultimate result that an increasing number of geriatric patients can be assisted to achieve the fullest participation in life within the limitation of their illness and disability. Medicare will generate the greatest preventive approach thus far to chronic disease control. It will facilitate the fusion of all the professional disciplines which assist in the total care of the aged patient. The provisions of this broad program will necessitate closer cooperation and cohesion between hospitals, physicians, skilled nursing homes, and home health agencies than has heretofore existed.

The sociological, psychological, and medical implications of this type of care were inconceivable prior to the conception of this legislation. The geriatric patient cannot help but benefit. Also, the record-keeping, the collating of information necessary to the administration of this broad program, will generate a vast reservoir of invaluable research material—data which will pinpoint the physical characteristics and medical syndromes of the older Americans.

In the future, hospitals will have extended care facilities located on their grounds and operate home health entities. The general hospital, nursing home, and home health components will be closely integrated and offer optimum supervision and potential of medical and health services.

> Such arrangements enable ailing elderly individuals to live out their days in such a nonhospital facility, with no greater dislocation or upset than possibly to move down a corridor or to a familiar nearby building for temporary periods of intermittent care or terminal care. In this way, all their needs can be met in a circumscribed familiar area which has become and will remain home to them for the rest of their days, without requiring extensive and disturbing, even terrifying, new arrangements and transfers. Examples of such ideal arrangements are existent and more can be anticipated. Two types may be cited: the sectarian, which is exemplified by the Swedish Convenant Home and Hospital and the Bethany Methodist Home and Hospital, both in Chicago; and the Federal Veterans Administration Centers, which also contain general hospitals, long-term care facilities, and domiciles (homes) combined under the same management and on the same grounds. Some of the Veterans Administration Centers are located in Milwaukee; Dayton; Kecoughton, Virginia; Bay Pines, Florida; and Los Angeles. As previously indicated, in these institutions, under one management and on the same familiar grounds, the domiciled resident may be easily transferred to the general hospital for diagnosis and acute treatment, then to the rehabilitation or convalescent facility, and finally back to the ambulant domicile. He may readily move back and forth between the various elements of the one facility, all well known to him, always having his requirements met in the unit which can best and most completely serve him.

The Administration on Aging is well aware that the new Medicare legislation will encounter many difficulties, some setbacks, and continued opposition from forces outside the Federal Government. It is the administration's sincere belief that eventually this piece of legislation will be a major step toward providing better health services for the aging. It will dispel the fear held by the majority of the elderly in the country with regard to the financial costs of chronic illnesses, hospitalization, and long-term care. It is also believed that a reduction of this apprehension on the part of the elderly will alleviate one of the major causes of mental disorders in this age group.

Chapter XIII

THE ROLE OF THE VOLUNTEER IN MAINTENANCE THERAPY

MARVIN S. ARFFA

THERE has been much recent publicity stressing the changing role of today's nursing home. New programs directed toward satisfying the unmet needs of aging persons, not previously given such attention, are being developed. The theme of this chapter is that effective use of volunteers from the community can be one essential ingredient in meeting the growing manpower and administrative crises facing these new programs which emphasize rehabilitation and maintenance therapy.

ROLE OF THE VOLUNTEER

Volunteers have played particular roles in national social welfare and health services for many years. As a distinct source of manpower, volunteers have performed services in neighborhood centers, youth agencies, hospitals, and in many other settings which would either have to hire people to perform services or forego services because of insufficient funds. Contributing significantly to the volume and quality of services provided through community agencies, they have played an important part of the total manpower team and can potentially be a greater part of this team in the fight against physical, psychological, and social deterioration in old age. Although the economic and productive values of volunteer service are most important, the greatest emphasis in developing volunteer opportunities might well be directed toward doing things *with* aging people rather than *for* them.

While volunteers are an important part of the therapeutic team, they serve in a complementary fashion and are not to be regarded as substitutes for other necessary personnel. Volunteers are often viewed as extensions of professional workers, reducing the burdens of understaffing and a heavy patient census. In fact, the manpower problem in the health-related disciplines has resulted in an expanding focus on the potential value of citizen volunteers or nonprofessionals as they are sometimes called. One consequence of this attention has been the formal training of a selected group of mature middle-class women to be mental health counselors. Emphasis on volunteer college students serving as companions to hospitalized chronic psychiatric patients is also noted.

The impact of the need for volunteer support in programs for the chronically ill has been further accentuated by an informal survey of nursing homes which revealed that only an average number of three hours per week for nurses and nine hours per week for aides were available for direct patient care. In a personal communication a leading physician who cares for stroke patients stated, "We have been most successful in rehabilitating stroke patients when we could initiate even a modest program within two weeks after the stroke and then progress from there." From a maintenance therapy point of view which demands large amounts of personal attention to patients at critical stages of chronicity, these findings have obvious and significant implications for the role of the volunteer in maintenance therapy.

One major role of the volunteer operates during the orientation process following admission to a long-term facility, whether it be a nursing home, convalescent home, or chronic disease hospital. Many patients coming to a long-term care facility experience the confusion of adapting to institutional living for the first time. Most of them are struggling to achieve emotional and social security. Therefore, the necessity for making further adjustments to their external environment, while at the same time seeking to make important inner adjustments, thrusts considerable strain upon them. If aging persons feel that they are alone in their doubts and insecurities, their problems are likely to become exaggerated. For this reason it is important to provide a sufficiently secure social setting where they can communicate freely about their difficulties. Providing companionship which paid personnel find difficult to give because of increasing lack of time as well as the nature of staff-patient relationships, volunteers help break down the barriers between the patient's isolation and the world of normal living.

One essential dimension of maintenance therapy is the development of a favorable emotional climate. Rudd and Margolin (1) state that "the creation of a favorable emotional climate . . . is conducive in encouraging the resident patients to participate willingly in routine as well as in maintenance activities." Patients tend to be sensitive to covert hostile attitudes which regular staff members may develop after prolonged exposure to periods of "no progress." The psychological support from volunteers who see residents as *people* rather than *patients* can have a profound effect on the morale of the total treatment milieu. The long-term facility is a functioning social institution and, as such, establishes the interdependence of patient behavior and social structure.

In a study by Beck, Kantor, and Gelineau (2), the impact of undergraduate volunteers on the social behavior of chronic psychotic patients was evaluated. They found that the introduction of volunteers modified the environment of the chronic patient so as to positively affect signs of withdrawal and desocialization, thereby increasing their social behavior. In another study, the same authors (3) found that 31 per cent of a group of 120 chronic psychotic patients were able to leave a chronic service following volunteer companion "treatment." The success of the program was attributed to 1) maintenance of a long period of volunteer-patient relationship, 2) flexibility of role definition for both volunteer and patient, and 3) volunteer activity extended beyond the hospital and into the community. The obvious assumption, then, is that one critical element in the development and maintenance of well-being is the daily association which patients have with persons who are concerned about them. The role which volunteers can play in this realm seems unique, invaluable, and irreplaceable.

Each resident in a nursing home or chronic disease setting must be expected, in terms of maintenance therapy, to live as active and full an existence as his current potential allows him. Rudd and Margolin (4) state that "maintenance therapy involves encouraging the patient, within his limitations, to enjoy to the fullest whatever life has to offer at his current physical or mental level." This paramount goal of preserving the existing level of function is not an easy task to accomplish. It implies some participation in activities, regardless of the functional level at which they are performed.

Mazer (5) suggested that volunteers provide the opportunities, the motivation, and the means for such participation. They provide opportunities by bringing in ideas, talents, and resources of the community; motivation by stimulating interest in the outside world and in other people; and the means by pushing the patient in a wheelchair, leading him by a steady hand, and encouraging him by a friendly voice. One example of an effective use of volunteers and community resources is demonstrated by a program in which volunteers, in cooperation with a local library, withdraw and deliver requested books to chronically disabled residents of nursing and convalescent homes. Thus, by bringing the outside world in, volunteers merge community resources with professional resources. Patients can identify and form relationships which are different from the relationships formed with staff members of the institution. While staff are doing all they can to help the patient within the limits of their time and energy, the volunteer contributes to the personal enhancement of the patient's activities of everyday living and to the maintenance of his roots in the community.

VOLUNTEER ACTIVITIES

The wide array of volunteer responsibilities can be generally designated as *patient-centered* and *administration-centered*.

Patient-centered

Patient-centered tasks usually involve direct patient contact, although not necessarily. These tasks are activities which essentially focus on the patient and his care. Assisting personnel to meet the individual needs of patients, volunteers may carry out a supervised nursing procedure and assist physicians, nurses, occupational therapists, physical therapists, exercise therapists, recreational therapists, and speech therapists with treatments or procedures. They may prepare and serve nourishment between meals. Patient-centered volunteers converse with patients; listen to their requests, wishes, and complaints; escort them within the setting and into the community; and perhaps teach them. They may make observations on the physical and psychological condition and behavior of patients, exchanging information with appropriate staff members. They may entertain and sponsor special projects.

The significance of patient-centered volunteer activities lies in the belief that "people need people." A human being must communicate with his fellow beings in order to be well and happy. Older people, in particular, need informal social relationships. Even if the older patient retains little or no residual handicaps from his disability, the fact that he is older, has been disabled, and has been separated from his familiar surroundings means that the continuity of his functioning within society has been interrupted. Much of the difficulty a patient has in maintaining contact with his social world revolves around the attitudes and expectations of others. His condition is likely to be uppermost in the thoughts of his family and friends. Instead of being regarded as a father, brother, husband, or employee, he is regarded as a patient in an "old folks" home.

Most important, he regards himself as a patient. Some research (6, 7) has suggested that the misconceptions and stereotypes which patients carry into nursing homes may affect their mortality potential. One implication of this finding is the individual's maintenance of the patient role, that is, the pattern of behaviors which the patient builds up in terms of what others expect or demand of him as a geriatric patient. This passive acceptance of the patient role impedes attempts at maintenance therapy. The factors of understaffing and impersonal professional relations also contribute to the maintenance of the patient role. These conditions partially account for the custodial orientation and atmosphere which pervade many nursing homes.

The goal of treating the patient or even that of meeting his basic physical needs often becomes obscured. In the custodial atmosphere the attitudes of staff and patients alike is one of control and avoidance of tension. While no one overtly resists patient improvement, quiet, passive, and cooperative behavior is rewarded and reinforced. The apparent ideal in this situation is the patient who necessitates no additional effort on the part of the staff. Volunteers can serve as buffers in this situation, breaking the patterns of underfunctioning and excessive dependency and lessening the shock of social disengagement through establishing meaningful interpersonal relationships. Volunteers often replace significant others in the individual's former life and become significant persons in his current life situation. They can explain and interpret to patients various management and treatment procedures, helping them to be less apprehensive and more amenable to treatment. Volunteers represent the concern of the community, and as peers in many instances, help to strengthen the individual's confidence and capacity to deal adequately with his environment and to manage his affairs within the limitations imposed upon him.

In relation to patient-centered volunteer activities, a recent article (8) specifically discussed volunteer services in convalescent hospitals, nursing homes, and homes for the aged in Oregon. It was reported that over two thousand volunteers have given service in these settings. Following the discovery that there was no organized framework for volunteer services in nursing homes, a survey was conducted to identify needs and potential resources. The survey committee found that in these homes,

> The residents had too much time on their hands and too little to do. Most people living there had little sociability, stimulation, or sympathetic companionship offered them. There seemed to be a vastly increased need for volunteer program and services to bridge the gap between the existing resources and the current needs of some of these older people. In spite of some unstructured volunteer services being given in a few places, generally activities were spotty, inadequate, or not at all. Such assistance for the most part still seemed to be almost in the process of discovery and development. In most locations there had been a failure to bring together

trained volunteers with organized programs of activity and the older people of these homes who at this time were so compellingly in need of certain help.

From the results of the survey emerged a pattern of an organized and coordinated program of a variety of volunteer services. The objective was "to provide satisfying and constructive activities to make their sunset years more bright and colorful and to add zest to their living through the concern, interest, and friendship from 'someone from the community who cares' . . . to increase communication and social interaction through the development of visitations, creative social and educational activities, and appropriate interest." Such service also assisted other professionals, for example, "When a volunteer brings a withdrawn, reserved geriatric person out of his shell so that he is better able to cooperate with the physical therapist, occupational therapist, et cetera."

Informal opinions indicate that in some nursing homes "the whole social climate has changed" as a result of the program.

> Residents are talking more with each other and wanting to give of themselves rather than being waited upon. Self-care has improved, and there is much better mental health, as many are more alert, with the senile patient less confused and cantankerous and more cooperative. Some patients are less irritable and less demanding and appear to have developed better attitudes and an ability to better accept their limitations and their situations. Many seem to have been brought out of their shells, to participate more, and appear happier. It is reported that a great number take more interest in their appearance and eat and sleep better, take less of the staff's time and have fewer psychosomatic complaints.

Administration-centered

The administration-centered volunteers, no less important than the patient-centered, are concerned with maintaining a safe and well-ordered environment and the managerial operations of the setting. Administration-centered tasks usually involve no patient contact. Volunteers may be involved in activities concerned with obtaining, dispensing, or maintaining materials and supplies for the setting. They may perform clerical activities such as assembling charts for new patients, checking charts, and copying records, or messenger activities such as delivering requisitions and picking up orders. They may also maintain rapport and promote good interpersonal relationships among staff, visitors, and others members of the community.

The significance of administration-centered activities is based on the impact of the total environment on the behavior and treatment of persons in long-term institutions (9, 10). Management in institutions has been visualized (11) as "that part of the process which relates to the creation of a positive or therapeutic learning environment wherein the activities described under the headings of evaluation and treatment are carried out." Management defined in this sense is regarded as a global concept which includes the general structuring of the environment in the service of the patient. "This might be the organizational structure of the hospital or ward including those administrative activities and attitudes which facilitate care and treatment, in addition to such things as the general psychological climate and the architecture of the building." Within this framework, volunteers are seen to "grease the wheels" of the institution's machinery which is necessary for the administration and effective operation of a physical setting conducive to therapeutic and maintenance therapies.

VOLUNTEER RECRUITMENT

Recruitment of volunteers can take place through local agencies such as employment services, public welfare agencies, schools, hospitals, neighborhood groups, church groups, and fraternal societies. Volunteers can be teenagers, college students, adults, and older or retired persons. They may come as members of an organized group or as individuals. There has been recent emphasis on having retired persons serve as volunteers in institutional settings. One unique program (12) was designed in Scranton, Pennsylvania, whereby older volunteers are trained to supervise therapeutic recreational activities for patients in four proprietary nursing homes. It was reported that forty-eight men and women, with a median age of sixty-eight years, were each assigned to a nursing home "to maintain consistency and continuity in relation to patients and personnel." This project verified the intuitive belief that "the well aging person is a prime resource for extending therapeutic recreation services to chronically ill or handicappd aging residents in a community's nursing homes."

SUMMARY

The role of volunteers in maintenance therapy may be viewed in relation to patients, to the long-term care facility, and to the community. In relation to patients, volunteers may provide them with orientation to their environment, encouraging them to meet personal needs through creation of a favorable emotional climate and by assisting in recreational and long-term rehabilitation therapies concerned with physical and psychological maintenance, and help them retain contact with their community. In relation to the long-term facility, volunteers can help supplement, complement, and stretch staff services to patients; share observations of patients with staff; and increase the staff's knowledge about the community and its potential resources. In relation to the community, volunteers can help develop cooperative relationships among community resources, help bridge the gap between the community and the facility by informing the community about the facility's activities, and help modify community attitudes toward aging persons in chronic disease and geriatric settings. In general, the kinds of activities beneficial to maintenance therapy which volunteers can perform are limited only by the imagination, creativity, and innovations of administrators and volunteer directors.

Volunteers fill specific needs, and a volunteer program should be well planned in advance to determine where the needs are and if volunteers can serve them. If such needs exist, then long-term care facilities without volunteer programs may be depriving their patients of an additional measure of care.

REFERENCES

1. RUDD, J. L., and MARGOLIN, R. J.: Maintenance therapy in physical medicine: relation to rehabilitation of the chronically ill. *J. Amer. Geriat. Soc.*, (June) 1964.

2. BECK, J. C.; KANTOR, D., and GELINEAU, V.: Impact of undergraduate volunteers on the social behavior of chronic psychotic patients. *Int. J. Soc. Psychiat., 11*:96-104, 1965.

3. BECK, J. C.; KANTOR, D., and GELINEAU, V.: Follow-up study of chronic psychotic patients "treated" by college case-aid volunteers. *Amer. J. Psychiat., 120*:269-271, 1963.

4. RUDD, J. L., and MARGOLIN, R. J.: Maintenance therapy in nursing homes. *Nurs. Home Admin.,* (November-December) 1965.

5. MAZER, J. L.: The volunteer in relation to activity programs for the institutionalized aged. *J. Amer. Geriat. Soc., 11*:607-611, 1963.

6. LIEBERMAN, M. A.: Relationships of mortality rates to entrance to a home for the aged. *Geriatrics, 16*:515, 1961.

7. FARRAR, M.; RYDER, M. B., and BLEUKNER, M.: Social work responsibility in nursing home care. *Social Casework, 45*:527-533, 1964.

8. PRAGOFF, M.: The volunteer program. *Oregon Health Bull., 44*:1-7, 1966.

9. STANTON, A. H., and SCHWARTZ, M. S.: *The Mental Hospitals.* New York, Basic Books, 1954.

10. CAUDILL, W.: *The Psychiatric Hospital as a Small Society.* Cambridge, Harvard, 1958.

11. ROSSBERG, R. H., and JACQUES, M. E.: The role of the group in patient evaluation, counseling and management. *Personnel and Guidance J., 40*:135-142, 1960.

12. *Volunteer Opportunities for Older Adults.* Memorandum 19, Committee on aging, Community Service Society of New York, Department of Public Affairs, 1965, pp. 30-31.

ADDENDUM

The following bibliography lists references related to using volunteers in medical and psychiatric settings which may be useful when considering the development of volunteer programs in maintenance therapy. The bibliography is divided into two sections: 1) Administration of Volunteer Programs, and 2) Volunteer Programs in Action. An additional section lists resources to whom inquiries about volunteer activities may be addressed.

Administration of Volunteer Programs

ACKERMAN, R. C.: How auxiliaries can keep pace. *Mod. Hosp., 80*:86, 1953.

Action for Mental Health: Final Report of the Joint Commission on Mental Illness and Health. New York, Basic Books, 1961, pp. 253-254.

Advisory council formed for volunteer program. *Ment. Hosp., 6*:22, 1965.

APPLE, D.: *Sociological Studies of Health and Sickness.* New York, Mc-Graw, 1960.

ARNETT, T. M.: Planning for the patient's discharge. *Mod. Hosp.*, 86:104-110, 1956.

AUBUCHON, M.: Role of the psychiatric volunteer. *Hosp. Prog.*, 43:142, 1962.

Auxiliaries and the American Hospital Association 1964 meeting, *Auxiliary Leader*, 5:1-6, 1964.

BECKER, D. G.: Exit lady bountiful: the volunteer and the professional social worker. *Social Service Review*, 38:57-72, 1964.

BLAIN, D., and TOMKINS, H. J.: Conference on volunteer services to psychiatric patients. *Ment. Hosp.*, 9:16-18, 1958.

BLAISDELL, R. E.: Institutional service unit movements. *Amer. J. Psychiat.*, 106:255-258, 1949.

BOLSTAD, G. L., and GINSBERG, S. T.: Volunteer services in state mental hospitals. *State Government*, 35:53-56, 1962.

BORKSTROM, E.: Planning and developing a volunteer service: basic principles. *Hospitals*, 28:74, 1954.

BOTTS, W. H.: Getting the volunteer program off to a good start. *Hospitals*, 33:43-44, 1959.

BRIDGES, J., and BEATRICE, M.: Volunteer workers in mental health. *Canad. Nurse*, 60:135-138, 1964.

BRIGHT, S.: Common factors in building understanding and broadening the base of citizen participation in health and welfare organizations. *Ment. Hyg.*, 37:30-35, 1953.

BROPHY, A.: Rehabilitation: a challenge to voluntary efforts. *Crippled Child*, 34:4-54, 1957.

BROWN, M. B.: What makes a successful director of volunteers? *Hosp. Manage.*, 80:60-62, 1955.

CARR, J. G.: Auxiliaries and volunteer services. *Hospitals*, 38:53-56, 1964.

CARTEY, K.: Orienting the hospital volunteer. *Ment. Hosp.*, 8:21, 1957.

CHERKASKEY, M.: The need for community planning for health care is today widely recognized. *Amer. J. Public Health*, 54:447-450, 1964.

CHURCH, D. M.: *How to Succeed with Volunteers.* New York, National P. R. Council of Health and Welfare Service, Inc., 1962.

COLEMAN, J. V.: Motivations of the volunteer in the health and welfare fields. *Ment. Hyg.*, 41:217-221, 1957.

Conference on development of standards and training curricula for volunteer services coordinators. *Psychiatric Studies and Projects*, 2, 1964.

Conference on volunteer services to psychiatric patients. *Ment. Hosp.*, 9:16-18, 1958.

CUMMING, E., and CUMMING, J.: *Closed Ranks: an Experiment in Mental Health Education.* Cambridge, Harvard, 1957.

DAVIES, I.: *Handbook for Volunteers in Mental Hospitals.* Minneapolis, U. of Minn., 1950.

DELANO, M. A.: Careful indoctrination needed for volunteers. *Ment. Hosp.,* 3:7, 1952.

DYKENS, W.: Recruiting mental hospital workers. *Ment. Hosp., 14:*538-540, 1963.

EWALT, J. R.: Volunteers. *In Mental Health Administration.* Springfield, Thomas, 1956, pp. 88-91.

FEBROW, G.: Evaluation of volunteers. *Hospitals, 36:*28, 1962.

FINN, T.: How to find new uses for volunteers. *AHA, Hospital Auxiliary Nursing League, 10:*4(a), 1958.

FINN, T.: New uses for volunteers. *AHA, Hospital Auxiliary Nursing League, 10:*4(b), 1958.

FLECK, S.: Recognition and utilization of the motivation of volunteers. *Ment. Hyg., 41:*222-227, 1957.

FORD, L. S.: Health and welfare workers—watch those peripheries. *Nurs. Outlook, 6:*564-565, 1958.

FRANK, M. H., and KILPATRICK, O.: *Volunteers in Mental Hospitals.* New York, National Association for Mental Health, 1955.

FRANK, M. H.: Hospital auxiliaries and volunteer service within hospitals. *Hospitals, 29:*448, 1955.

GEE, A. M.: The mental hospital and volunteer programs. *Ment. Hosp.,* 9:38-41, 1958.

GREENBLATT, M.; YORK, R., and BROWN, E. L.: *From Custodial to Therapeutic Care in Mental Hospitals.* New York, Russell Sage, 1955.

GREENBLATT, M.: A Role of the Voluntary Organizations in the Work of Mental Institutions. Paper read at American Association of University Women, Boston, 1957.

GREENBLATT, M.: The volunteer in the community-expanding opportunities. In *The Volunteer and the Psychiatric Patient.* Natalie D. Spingarn (Ed.), Washington, D. C., American Phychiatric Association, 1959.

Guidelines for use of volunteers in departments of social work in hospitals: American Hospital Association statement. *Hospitals, 37:*95, 1963.

HIXSON, H. H.: The director of volunteers as a department head. *Hospitals,* 38:64-67, 1964.

Hospital Auxiliaries and Volunteers. Report of a survey conducted by the American Hospital Association, 1963.

Hospitals Volunteer Services. Chicago, AHA, 1954.

Interim Report of the Committee on Volunteer Service in Hospitals. Chicago, AHA, 1958.

JANDA, E. M.: Orientation and training: pinpointing the differences. *Auxiliary Leader, 4:*1-6, 1963.

KIMBALL, J.: *Guide for Organization of Volunteer Services in Mental Hospitals.* Massachusetts Association for Mental Health, 1950.

KIRSHMAN, E.: Volunteer and the human condition. *Ment. Hosp.,13:*265, 1962.

Lets Measure Up—A Set of Criteria for Evaluating a Volunteer Program.

The Volunteer Bureau, United Community Services of Metropolitan Boston, January, 1962.

LUIN, L.: *A Handbook of Hospital Psychiatry: A Practical Guide to Therapy.* New York, Int. Univs., 1955, Ch. 13.

McBEE, M., and FRANK, M.: *Volunteer Participation in Psychiatric Hospital Services.* New York, National Committee for Mental Hygiene, 1950.

MACKIN, M. C., and JONES, L. P.: Youth wants to serve. *Ment. Hosp.,* 12:14-17, 1961.

MARTIN, D. H.: Individual orientation for volunteers. *Ment. Hosp.,* 6:23, 1955.

MILNE, J.: Voluntary service and the mental hospital. *Ment. Hosp.,* 8:64-70, 1956.

Orientation and indoctrination of volunteer workers in VA hospitals. *Veterans Administration Technical Bulletin,* 6:28, 1947.

PAPIER, S.: Directing a volunteer program. *Hosp. Manage.,* 88:42-43, 1959.

PARKE, J. H.: Judging a volunteer program means judging its director. *Hospitals,* 33:44-46, 1959.

PRATT, S., *et al.*: Role of the mental hospital volunteer, in "The Mental Hospital and the 'Treatment Field'." *Psychol. Studies,* 11:162-179, 1960.

RANDOLPH, A. K.: Warning: volunteer shortage ahead. *Hospitals,* 38:63-64, 1964.

SAUNDERS, M.: "How" you begin is important. *Hosp. Manage.,* 79:47-48, 1955.

SAUNDERS, M.: Putting a volunteer program in action. *Hosp. Manage.,* 80:46, 1955.

SCHILLER, M. M. B.: Volunteers—asset or anathema? *Mod. Hosp.,* 56:73-74, 1941.

SCHUMAKER, C. J., JR.: Volunteer auxiliaries and hospital prestige. *Hosp. Manage.,* 97:59-62, 1964.

Screening of VA volunteer hospital workers. *Veterans Administration Technical Bulletin,* 6:47, 1948.

SEATON, M.: Uncovering the costs of volunteer turnover. *Auxiliary Leader,* 5:1-5, 1964.

Selecting volunteers for the psychiatric services. *Auxiliary Leader,* 5:1-5, 1964.

SHARPE, A. A.: Why volunteers in Illinois mental hospitals? *Welfare Bulletin,* Springfield, Illinois Department of Public Welfare, 1952.

SHARPE, A. A.: *How Volunteers Work in State Hospitals.* State of Illinois, Department of Public Welfare, 1953.

SILLS, D.: The volunteers. (bd. rev.), *Nurs. Outlook,* 7:129, 1959.

SMITH, J. A.: Selecting volunteers for the psychiatric service. *Auxiliary Leader,* 5:1-5, 1964.

SPINGARN, N. D., (Ed.): *The Volunteer and the Psychiatric Patient.* Washington, D. C., American Psychiatric Association, 1959.

Status of the director of volunteer service. *AHA, Hospital Auxiliary Nursing League, 10*:4, 1958.

STUBBS, M.: Volunteers in the vocational rehabilitation program. *Rehab. Rec., 4*:7-8, 1963.

Teenage Volunteer in the Hospital. Chicago, AHA, 1962.

The Volunteer and the Psychiatric Patient. Washington, American Psychiatric Association, 1959.

THURSZ, D.: Past relic or future asset? *Rehab. Rec., 4*:3-6, 1963.

THURSZ, D.: Volunteers: past relic or future assets? *Hosp. Topics, 42*:23-24, 1964.

Use of Volunteers in Public Welfare. New York, Family Service Association of America, 1963.

Utilization of volunteer services in VA hospitals. *Veterans Administration Technical Bulletin, 6*:29, 1947.

VAN, G. P.: Recommended: a salaried director of volunteers. *Canad. Hosp., 41*, 1964.

Volunteer Participation in Psychiatric Hospital Services: Organization Manual and Program Guide. New York, The National Committee for Mental Hygiene, 1950.

Volunteer workers needed. *Occup. Outlook Quart., 8*:30, 1964.

VON MERING, O.: The social self-renewal of the mental patient and the volunteer movement. In *The Patient and the Mental Hospital.* M. Greenblatt, D. J. Levinson and R. H. Williams (Eds.), New York, Free Press of Glencoe, Inc., 1957.

VON MERING, O., and KING, S. H.: Social self-renewal and community volunteers. In *Remotivating the Mental Patient,* New York, Russell Sage 1957, pp. 155-180.

What kind of person should the volunteer director be? *AHA, Hospital Auxiliary Nursing League, 10*:4, 1958.

WHITE, H. F., JR.: Strengths and weaknesses of volunteers and volunteers systems. *Mod. Hosp., 80*:98-102, 1953.

Working With Volunteers. Leadership Pamphlet 10, Adult Education Association, 1956.

Volunteer Programs in Action

Achievement awards, 1963: bronze award—Camarillo State Hospital. *Ment. Hosp., 14*:532-533, 1963.

Albany teens are stars in stripes. *Nurs. Outlook, 6*:517, 1958.

ALEXANDER, J.: They "doctor" one another. *Saturday Evening Post,* December 6, 1952.

ARMSTRONG and BURCHARDT: When disaster strikes, *Amer. Ass. Indust. J., 8*:26-27, 1960.

A summer work experience: a pilot program in recruitment for a mental health career. Mental Health Association of Houston and Harris County, (Texas Association for Mental Health), September, 1963.

Auxiliary volunteers help with activities. *Ment. Hosp., 3*:6, 1952.

BAILEY, N. F.: When the students volunteered. *Ment. Hosp., 13*:469, 1962.

BAKER, E.: Operation Bunny Rabbit. *Auxiliary Leader, 5*:14-15, 1964.

BARTHOLOMEW, A. A., and KELLEY, M. F.: Personal emergency advisory service. *Ment. Hyg., 46*:382-392, 1962.

BAYER, M. E.: Volunteers and senior citizens. *Recreation Magazine,* March, 1962.

BEERS, P.: Teen-age volunteers at state school. *Ment. Hosp., 14*:447, 1963.

BENNETT, E.: Teen-agers train for community service. *Volta Review,* 67:228-229, 1965.

BERRY, E.: Volunteer program penetrates a maximum security setting. *Ment. Hosp., 14*:503, 1963.

BIRD, E. S., and KNAPP, S. E.: Volunteers in government hospitals. *Southern Hosp., 11*:29, 1963.

BRUCE, T. C.: Want a good job with no pay? *Recreation Magazine,* October, 1951.

BUTTS, B.: A panhandler. *Recreation Magazine,* October, 1953.

CALLAGHAN, T. P.: Candy striper contributes valuable time and talents. *Southern Hosp., 30*:38, 1962.

CALVERT, R., JR., and KENNEDY, P. M.: Career assistance for returning Peace Corps volunteers. *The Personnel and Guidance J., 43*:447-450, 1965.

CAMERON, D. C.: Honorable mention: Minnesota Department of Public Welfare. *Ment. Hosp., 9*:20-22, 1958.

Candy stripers. *Ment. Hosp., 14*:646, 1963.

CARLETTI, J. A.: Volunteers provide companionship therapy under social service supervision. *Ment. Hosp., 15*:691-693, 1964.

CARSON, C.: Red Cross youth volunteers program at Heritage of Edina. *Nurs. Home, 12*:7, 1963.

CARTER, M. G.: Youth participation in community mental health program. *Ment. Hyg., 35*:581-588, 1951.

Children's Care Committee Service in London—a review of the last 10 years. *Brit. J. Nurs., 104*:29-31, 1956.

Christmas 'round the calendar. *Ment. Hosp., 13*:657, 1962.

Church group aids special project. *Ment. Hosp., 5*:17, 1954.

Citizen participation. *Recreation Magazine,* April, 1954.

CLANCY, S.: Bathtime at St. Mary's. *Catholic Nurse, 10*:34-37, 1962.

College girls perform varied services. *Ment. Hosp., 7*:20, 1956.

COLLINS, J. W.: They also serve who have retired. *Mod. Hosp., 84*:85-86, 1955.

Cookie-baking sessions for neuropsychiatric patients. *Auxiliary Leader,* 3:15, 1962.

Cox, C.: Nurses' aides in bobby socks. *Registered Nurse,* 19:66-67, 1956.

CRANE, J.: What my junior volunteer work means to me. *Auxiliary Leader,* 5:14-15, 1964.

CROLL, B.: A women's auxiliary in action. *Canad. Nurse,* 52:25-26, 1956.

CZATT, M.: Volunteer guild as asset to private hospital. *Ment. Hyg.,* 4:15, 1953.

DALAMAS, H.: The act nobody can buy. *Recreation Magazine,* June, 1952.

DARNTON, P. H.: Volunteers in a large hospital. *Hosp. Manage.,* 87:52, 1959.

DAUNCEY, H. M.: Using volunteers in a recreation program. *Recreation Magazine,* December, 1951.

DeLISSOVOY, V.: Increasing the "psychological income" of the hospital volunteer. *Hosp. Manage.,* 97:88-92, 1964.

DENNINGER, J.: They ease the nursing shortage. *Today's Health,* 36:38-39, 1958.

DePRANO, J. E.: Volunteer workers in a creation program. *Recreation Magazine,* December, 1956.

DIETZ, J.: Ten colleges participate in new mental health course. *The Boston Globe,* September, 1964, p. 13.

DOHAN, J. L.: Development of a student program in a state mental hospital. In *The Patient and the Mental Hospital.* M. Greenblatt, D. J. Levinson, and R. H. Williams (Eds.), New York, Free Press of Glencoe, Inc., 1957, pp. 593-603.

DOUDS, D. V.: Nursing for the love of it. *Registered Nurse,* 21:70-72, 1958.

DUBROW, M.; NITZBERG, J., and TOBIAS, J.: Unpaid workers and retarded youth. *Rehab. Rec.,* 4:9-13, 1963.

DUDLEY, M.: How volunteers are easing the nurse's load. *Registered Nurse,* 22:35-39, 1959.

DWYER, T. E.: Any veteran will tell you—volunteers make a good hospital. *Mod. Hosp.,* 82:92-96, 1954.

ELIASOPH, E.: The use of volunteers as case aides in a treatment setting. *Social Casework,* 40:141-144, 1959.

ESLICK, H.: Training instructs. *Auxiliary Leader,* 4:1-6, 1963.

EVANS, R. L.: Volunteers in mental hospitals. *Ment. Hyg.,* 39:111-117, 1955.

EWALT, P. L.: Massachusetts introduces students to mental health careers. *Ment. Hosp.,* 16:212-213, 1965.

FAY, E., and LEE, T.: Let's look at volunteer service. *Brit. Med. Quart.,* 7:122-124, 1956.

FECHNER, A. H., and PARKE, J. H.: Volunteer worker and the psychiatric hospital. *Amer. J. Psychiat.,* 107:602-606, 1951.

FELDMAN, H. W.: Student companions for mental patients. *Public Health Rep.,* 77:410, 1962.

FELDMAN, H. W.: College Students as Volunteer Companions in a Mental

Hospital. (Mimeograph), Topeka, Veterans Administration Hospital, August, 1961.

FELLOWS, W. M.: Study of participation of youth in volunteer service to VA hospitals. *Planning Letter No. 57-27,* Veterans Administration, Washington, D. C.

FERRIS, P. D.: Boy Scout volunteers. *Auxiliary Leader,* 3:13-14, 1962.

FISHER, C. E.: Volunteer participation in home finding in the foster home care program. *United States Veterans Administration Program Guide,* 10:14-16, 1956.

FOVAL, R. J.: Adult recreation clubs. *Recreation Magazine,* March, 1953.

FRAKES, R. A.: The Harper Hospital Auxiliary. *Nurs. Outlook,* 10:326-327, 1962.

FRANK, M. H.: Volunteers in mental hospitals. *Ment. Hyg.,* 32:411-423, 1948.

FRANK, M. H.: Volunteer work with psychiatric patients. *Ment. Hyg.,* 33:353-365, 1949.

GALATZAN, L.: 24 in white. *Texas Hosp.,* 18:8-9, 1962.

GALLAGHER, P.: Selecting community leaders. *Recreation Magazine,* February, 1951.

GAMBLE, J. D.: New frontier in hospitals. *Hosp. Prog.,* 44:83, 1963.

GATES, S.: Community leaders use your initiative. Recreation *Magazine,* March, 1952.

GLASMANN, R.: Hidden assets: a youth volunteer program in a psychiatric hospital. *Bedford Research,* 9, VA Hospital, Bedford, 1963.

GOLDSMITH, N.: Volunteer program helps teen-agers find careers in the health field. *Mod. Hosp.,* 100:6-7, 1963.

GOLDSTEIN, S., and BENEDICT, L.: Use of volunteers in a home care program. *Hosp. Manage.,* 97:52-54, 1964.

GOLL: Just 10 minutes more. *Crippled Child,* 34:12, 1957.

GRANT, L. A.: "Flashdrive" pays off. *Recreation Magazine,* May, 1951.

Grant for conference on volunteers. *Ment. Hosp.,* 8:21, 1957.

GREENBLATT, M., and KANTOR, D.: Student volunteer movement and the manpower shortage. *Amer. J. Psychiat.,* 118:809-814, 1962.

GROSS, A.: Teen-age volunteer—Vicki's two faces. *Auxiliary Leader,* 3:1-6, 7-11, 1962.

HADDOCK, J. N., and DUNDON, H. D.: Volunteer work in a state hospital by college students. *Ment. Hyg.,* 35:599-603, 1951.

HALL, B. B., and LAFAVE, H. G.: Volunteers with special skills supplement professionals at state hospital. *Hosp. Topics,* 41:43, 1963.

HALL, C. W.: America's amazing woman. *Reader's Digest,* July, 1955.

HERTZ, B. V.: Let's help teen-agers open doors to useful vocations. *Auxiliary Leader,* 3:1-6, 1962.

HEYD, E. H.: Through teen-age program, hospitals have advantage in current competition for the best personnel. *Southern Hosp.,* 30:31-32, 1962.

HICKEY, M.: New York City's privileged teen-agers. *Ladies' Home Journal*, 79:6, 1962.

HOLZBERG, J. D.: The companion program: implementing the manpower recommendations of the Joint Commission on Mental Illness and Health. *Amer. Psychol.*, 18:224-226, 1963.

HOLZBERG, J. D.: *The Significance of the Companionship Experience for the College Student*. Washington, D. C., United States Government Printing Office, 1964.

HOLZBERG, J. D., and KNAPP, R. H.: The social interaction of college students and chronically ill patients. *Amer. J. Orthopsychiat.*, 34:487-492, 1964.

HOLZBERG, J. D.; WHITTING, H. S., and LOURY, D. G.: Chronic patients and a college companion program. *Ment. Hosp.*, 15:152-158, 1964.

HOMAN, A.: Volunteers assist with visitors. *Ment. Hosp.*, 7:22, 1956.

HOOVER, C. A.: Role of the auxiliary in the hospital's public relations is important. *AHA, Hospital Auxiliary Nursing League*, 10:3, 1958.

HORCHOW, F., and KEMP, M. B.: To tell the public, sell them. *Nurs. Outlook*, 5:296-299, 1957.

How candy stripers earn their stars. *Mod. Hosp.*, 98:93-95, 1962.

How teen-agers can help in the medical record department. *Auxiliary Leader*, 3:14-15, 1962.

HUDSON, E. L.: The therapy of friendliness. *J. Amer. Geriat.*, 11:496-504, 1963.

HUGHES, N.: Volunteers in VA hospitals believe in the practical application of altruism. *Mod. Hosp.*, 78:90-92, 1952.

HULSBIZER, E.: Carolers sing for everyone. *Recreation Magazine*, December, 1954.

HYDE, R. W., and HURLEY, C. F.: Volunteers in mental hospitals. *Psychiat. Quart. [Suppl.]*, 24:233-249, 1950.

If you ask me. *Amer. J. Nurs.*, 57:317, 1957.

JEROME, A., and REID, M.: Ladies who listen. *Nurs. Outlook*, 5:216-218, 1957.

JOHNSON, B. F.: The children find fun and health in pediatrics program. *Mod. Hosp.*, 92:90-91, 1959.

JOHNSTON, A.: Help for the home bound. *Recreation Magazine*, 49:388-389, 1956.

JORDHEIM, A.: The health activities of Norwegian women. *Nurs. Outlook*, 4:106-108, 1956.

Judge sentences speeders to hospital volunteer work. *Public Relations News Letter*, October, 1962.

Junior Aides lend a hand. *Practical Nurs.*, 7:11, 1957.

Junior Corps at Morristown Memorial: a group of teen-age boys who want to do "something worthwhile." *Hosp. Topics*, 40:40, 1962.

KANTOR, D.: The use of college students as case aides in a social service department of a state hospital: an experiment in undergraduate social work education. In *The Patient and the Mental Hospital.* M. Greenblatt, D. J. Levinson and R. H. Williams (Eds.), New York, Free Press of Glencoe, Inc., pp. 603-608.

KANTOR, D.: Inducing preferences for mental health careers. *Monograph 75, National Association of Social Workers,* October, 1959.

KANTOR, D. B., and GREENBLATT, M.: Wellmet: halfway to community rehabilitation. *Ment. Hosp., 13:*146-152, 1962.

KARLINS, M. M.: Volunteers in state mental hospitals. *Nurs. Outlook, 2:*264, 1954.

KARLINS, M.: Use of volunteers in mental hospitals. *Ment. Hosp., 5:*8, 1954.

KECK, A.: One dose per syringe. *Nurs. Outlook, 7:*24-25, 1959.

Kid sister volunteers. *Auxiliary Leader, 5:*8-109, 1964.

KILPATRICK, A.: Foundation sponsors pilot volunteer projects. *Ment. Hosp., 6:*6-8, 1955.

KING, S. T.: Beauty treatments help mentally ill. *Red Cross Courier, 42:*14-15, 1950.

KIRK, W. R.: Hard-working ambassadors merge hospital community aims. *Hospitals, 33:*52-53, 1959.

KLEIN, W. L., and ZAX, M.: The use of a hospital volunteer program in the teaching of abnormal psychology. *J. Soc. Psychol., 65:*155-165, 1965.

KLINENS, N. S.: Volunteer workers. *Occup. Ther. Rehab., 26:*153-166, 1947.

KLUGMAN, S. F., and KLUGMAN, C. H.: High school volunteers find summer work rewarding. *Ment. Hosp., 15:*274-275, 1964.

KRAFT, I.: The Use of Volunteers as Social Work Technicians in a Child Psychiatry Clinic. Paper read at American Orthopsychiatric Association meeting, 1965.

KRAVITZ, S., and LAMBERT, C., JR.: Volunteer interviewers among the elderly. *Gerontologist, 3:*55-60, 90, 1963.

KRUSE, A. H.: The outlook for voluntary social work services. *Social Work, 31:*27-32, 1950.

KURLAND, A. A.: In praise of volunteers. *Ment. Hyg., 39:*350, 1955.

KYLES, J. A.: Staff boss for willing workers. *Canad. Hosp., 41:*41, 1964.

LANGDON, D. T.: Volunteers in a crippled children's program. *Community Health Bull., 66:*35-38, 1952.

LAWTON, M., and LIPTON, M. B.: Student employees become companions to patients. *Ment. Hosp., 14:*550-556, 1953.

LEE, D. T.: New dimensions for volunteers. *Ment. Hyg., 46:*273-282, 1962.

LIBBY, E.: Estimating volunteer's payroll. *Hosp. Manage., 97:*96-97, 1964.

LICHTENBERG, B.: On the selection and preparation of the Big Brother volunteer. *Social Casework, 37:*396-400, 1956.

LOCKE, H. J.: Are volunteer interviewees representative? *Social Problems, 1:*143-146, 1954.

LONGENECHER, F. R.: Delaware's auxiliary sets precedent in hospital-community relations. *Ment. Hosp., 7,* 1956.

LUCCHESI, P. F.: Health careers recruitment. *Hospitals,* 37:36, 1963.

MACBAIN, N., and SCHUMACHER, L.: Premedical students learn hospital routine as volunteers. *Hospitals,* 37:73-75, 1963.

MACPHEE, J. A., and FOWLER, V. L.: Let's use college volunteers. *Recreation Magazine,* January, 1954.

McCANN, W. H.: Psychologists discover value of volunteers. Volunteers learn test techniques. *Ment. Hosp., 15:*269-271, 1964.

McCLORY, H.: Volunteer aids for problem-ridden families. *Children,* 8:175-178, 1961.

McGRIFF, D. L.: A volunteer program in a neuropsychiatric hospital. *Social Casework,* 37:29-33, 1956.

MAGNUSSEN, A. A., and POPKIN, R.: On the Red Cross centenary—nurses join in the observance in their work around the world. *Amer. J. Nurs.,* 63:75-77, 1963.

MALAMUD, I. T.: Volunteers in community mental health work. *Ment. Hyg.,* 39:300-309, 1955.

Male volunteers work at VA hospitals. *Ment. Hosp.,* 4:6, 1953.

Manitoba Women's Hospital Auxiliaries Association. *Canad. Nurse.,* 56:138-141, 1960.

MARK, A. H.: Men of mercy lighten the load. *Mod. Hosp.,* 86:88-92, 1956.

MARKOWITZ, R., and STEIN, F.: Volunteers become involved in health careers. *Hosp. Manage.,* 94:36-37, 1962.

MARQUIS, J. G.: An Experiment in Changing Employer Attitudes toward Mental Illness: the "X" Factor in Community Programs on the Employment of Former Patients. Unpublished manuscript presented at the meeting of the National Association of Mental Health, November 22, 1957.

MAUKSCH, I.: Wanted: volunteers for research. *Nurs. Outlook, 12:*69-70, 1964.

MAY, D. C.: The use of volunteers in conjunction with psychotherapy. *Smith College Studies in Social Work,* 20:173-189, 1950.

MAZER, J. L.: The volunteer in relation to activity programs for the institutionalized aged. *J. Amer. Geriat. Soc.,* 11:607-611, 1963.

MENDTE, J. R.: Little Miriams do a big job. *Hosp. Progr.,* 44:84-85, 1963.

Men's guide appeals for more volunteers. *Ment. Hosp.,* 3:11, 1952.

MILLER, E. A.: Patients like the "charm class." *Ment. Hosp.,* 7:8, 1956.

MILTON, H.: Candy striper is not a masculine term. *Auxiliary Leader,* 3:7, 1962.

MILNE, J.: Community participation in the mental hospitals. *Ment. Health,* 11:66-69, 1952.

MILTON, H. E.: Auxiliaries and volunteer service. *Hospitals,* 33:45-47, 1959.

MITCHELL, W.: Fictive Siblings and the "Unworthy Child" in Changing

Rural Vermont. (Mimeograph), Montpelier, The Hope Foundation, 1965.

MOORE, B. M.: *Volunteer Services—Modern "Miracle."* Austin, Hogg Foundation, 1958.

MOORE, M.: Activities of a junior board of directors. *Recreation Magazine,* November, 1951.

MOTT, B. D.: Young citizens improve recreation areas. *Recreation Magazine,* June, 1957.

MULANEY, G.: Voluntary service in an official agency. *Nurs. Outlook,* 5:141-154, 1957.

MURRAY, J. F.: Community services program at Agnews State Hospital. *Dis. Nerv. Sys.,* 14:242-246, 1955.

NEISSER, E. G.: Citizens of the middle years: the pick of the volunteer crop. *Blueprint for Health,* 17:16-19, 1963.

NILLSON, G. L.: Citizen volunteers in the cause of mental health. *Ment. Hyg.,* 35:373-385, 1951.

Operation kindness. *The American Child,* Washington, D. C., National Committee on Employment of Youth, March, 1962.

Our volunteers. *Maryland Soc. Med. J.,* 11:112, 1962.

OVERHOLSER, W.: The volunteer in psychiatric rehabilitation. *Ment. Hyg.,* 45:163-166, 1961.

PACE, B.: Teen-age volunteers in Austin State School. *Texas Hosp.,* 18:13, 1962.

PALMER, M.: Report on Experiment with Two Volunteers. Unpublished report, Massachusetts Mental Health Center, 1956.

PARKE, J. H.: Cost of free service. *Ment. Hosp.,* 4:11, 1953.

PARKE, J. H.: Enlisting retired elderly persons for volunteer service. *Hospitals,* 38:67-68, 1964.

PARKER, C.: Nursing at a career-o-rama. *Nurs. Outlook,* 8:79, 1960.

Partners on the job. *Recreation Magazine,* May, 1950.

PATTEN, E. B.: Unique junior program—music therapy. *Texas Hosp.,* 18:12, 1963.

Peace Corps is psychiatric success. *U. S. Med.,* 1:30-31, 1965.

PERKINS, N.: Volunteer workers in mental hospitals. *Nurs. Outlook,* 7:288-290, 1959.

PHELAN, E. J.: The Anthonettes: girls on the "go." *Hosp. Progr.,* 44:86-88, 1963.

PINANSKI, V.: New trends in training volunteers. *Mod. Hosp.,* 88:86, 1957.

Placing volunteers. *Recreation Magazine,* May, 1954.

POSER, E. G.: Volunteers in mental hospitals. *Canad. Ment. Health,* 11:29-31, 1963.

PRATT, S. SCOTT, G.; TREESH, E.; KHANNA, J.; LESHER, T.; GARDINER, G., and WRIGHT, W.: Exploration of Selected Aspects of the (Mental Hospitals) Staff-Patient-Town Configuration. Proposal for a group research project, unpublished prospectus, Formed (Kansas) State Hospital, 1960.

RANDOLPH, A. K.: Developing ample volunteer resources. *Auxiliary Leader*, 5:1-6, 1964.

RAPPAPORT, J.: Homecoming: a volunteer program. *Perspect. Psychiat. Care*, 11:41-45, 1964.

RAUCK, M.: From consultant to owner. *Nurs. Outlook*, 7:152-153, 1959.

REARDON, D.: A community takes a hand. *Recreation Magazine*, April, 1951.

REBBOLZ, M. T.: Day camp program for "why-daddies." *Recreation Magazine*, May, 1955.

REED, C. E.: The need for more lay interest. *Recreation Magazine*, October, 1953.

REICHENBERG-HACKETT, W.: Senior citizens in community work. *Ment. Hyg.*, 39:574-580, 1955.

REINHERZ, H.: Leadership of student volunteers. *Ment. Hosp.*, 13:600, 1962.

REINHERZ, H.: College student volunteers as case aides in a state hospital for children. *Amer. J. Orthopsychiat.*, 33:544-546, 1963.

Reporter's notebook. *Recreation Magazine*, February, 1957.

REYNOLDS, H.: Nurses shaped this volunteer program. *Hospitals*, 33:47, 1959.

REYNOLDS, H. L.: Information center acquaints teen-agers with hospital career opportunities. *Auxiliary Leader*, 4:10-12, 1963.

RICK, T. A.; GILMORE, A. S., and WILLIAMS, C. F.: Volunteer work with the mentally retarded. *Rehab. Rec.*, 5:4-6, 1964.

RIDGEWAY, E. P.: Volunteer program at Delaware State Hospital. *Amer. J. Occup. Ther.*, 54:205-206, 1951.

RIFE, M.: An old house comes to life. *Recreation Magazine*, November, 1955.

ROBSON, M. I. M.: Meals on wheels, *Nurs. Times*, 55:928, 1959.

ROOD, A. C.: Auxiliaries answer the challenge of mental hospital service: understanding opens doors. *Hospitals*, 29:70-71, 1955.

ROSS, L.: Our planning extends beyond the discharge date. *Hospitals*, 30:37-38, 1956.

SANBORN, E.: Recognition for volunteer service. *Hospitals*, 29:40, 1955.

SAUCIER, D. S., and HODA, P.: Patients help patients. *Ment. Hosp.*, 11:57, 1960.

SAUNDERS, M.: Teen-agers take to hospital work. *Mod. Hosp.*, 91:76-77, 1958.

SCHMITZ, M. E.: The use of volunteers in case work. *The Family*, 24:50-57, 1944.

SCHOEN, K. F.: Nursery solves baby-sitting problem for volunteers. *Ment. Hosp.*, 14:293, 1963.

SCHULENBURG, D. E.: Connecticut Service Corps: Summer, 1964. Unpublished report, Norwich Hospital, Connecticut State Department of Mental Health, 1965.

SCHULHOFER, E.: Agency experience for the preprofessional student. *J. Social Casework, 30*:196-200, 1949.

Scouts cheer patients with tray favors. *Hospitals, 36*:23-24, 1962.

SEEL, D. W.: The story of a charm class. *Recreation Magazine,* September, 1955.

SHARP, J. A.: Father on the playground. *Recreation Magazine,* September, 1951.

SHAW, H. F.: Volunteers take a look at themselves. *Ment. Hosp., 11*:40-42, 1960.

SHOEMAKER, R., and BIGELOW, E.: The disappearing playroom. *Nurs. Outlook, 7*:156-158, 1959.

SHORE, H.: How to get better results with volunteers. *Nurs. Home, 5*:16, 1963.

SHRIVER, R. S.: A new breed of American. *Occup. Outlook Quart., 8*:1-4, 1964.

SHUMAN, I.: Expatients make good volunteers. *Ment. Hosp., 11*:28-29, 1960.

SILLS, D. H.: *Volunteers in Social Service.* New York, National Travelers Aid Association, 1947, pp. 1-51.

SILSON, J. E.; ELLIOTT, C. M., and BEATRICE, H. H.: *Recreation in Hospitals.* New York, National Recreation Association, 1959.

SILVER, S.: Recreation workshop. *Recreation Magazine,* November, 1952.

SIMONSON, L.: Snake-pit volunteers. *Christian Advocate,* 1952, pp. 127-135.

SIMPSON, V. R.: The Chaplain and Program of Religious Education Using College Volunteers. Presented to the Chaplain Section, American Association on Mental Deficiency, June 10, 1965.

SIMS, N. J.: Volunteers in social work. *Social Work Yearbook,* 1951, pp. 537-542.

SMITH, H. D.: Volunteer program in Illinois mental hospitals. *Public Aid in Illinois, 19*:4, 1952.

SNYDER, R. M.: A volunteer program for older persons. *Recreation Magazine,* December, 1954.

SPEARE: Don't shut out the shut-ins. *Crippled Child, 34*:20-25, 1956.

SPENCE, H.: The mental patients' best friends. *Saturday Evening Post,* June 19, 1954.

State volunteer program expanded in Minnesota. *Ment. Hosp., 5*:11, 1954.

STETSON, E. R.: Role played by volunteers in a mental hospital. *Amer. J. Occup. Ther., 5*:203, 1951.

STEVENSON, G. S.: Dynamic considerations in community functions. *Ment. Hyg., 34*:531-546, 1950

STEVENSON, G. S.: A mental health program for lay groups. *Bull. World Fed. Ment. Health, 2*:14-18, 1950.

STIERILI, D. M.: An astronomy group. *Recreation Magazine,* November, 1950.

STOBBE, P. T.: Have an all-sports night. *Recreation Magazine,* October, 1955.

STOHLER, E. H.: Outstanding volunteer service program in a community hospital. *Southern Hosp., 23*:26, 1955.

STRIVER: Nurses galore. *Nurs. Times, 57*:744-745, 1961.

STUBBS, M.: Volunteers in the vocational rehabilitation program. *Rehab. Rec., 4*:7-9, 1963.

SUGARMAN, P., and FINER, N. S.: Volunteers can humanize patient care. *Hospitals, 27*:89-90, 1953.

SUSSMAN, P.: Teen-age volunteers. *Hospitals, 33*:14, 1959.

SUSSMAN, P.: How young a volunteer? *Hospitals, 36*:26, 1962.

SUSSMAN, P. Youth activity programs. *Hospitals, 37,* 1963.

SWAN, H. T.: Reno's clown alley. *Recreation Magazine.* January, 1951.

TAYLOR, F., and BAIRD, E.: A perfect fit for the volunteer program. *Hospitals, 31*:33-35, 1957.

Teen-agers help the handicapped. *Auxiliary Leader, 5*:7-8, 1964.

Teen-age volunteers aid physicians in unusual program for mentally ill. *JAMA, 189*:41, 1964.

Teen-age volunteer program: Morristown, New Jersey Memorial Hospital. *Prof. Nurs. Home, 4*:4, 1962.

Teen-age volunteers are unqualified success at the Veterans Administration 169 hospitals. *Southern Hosp., 30*:54, 1962.

The debt we owe to the volunteers. *Life and Health, 74*:8, 1959.

The human side. *Nurs. Outlook, 8*:421, 1960.

The Voluntary Service Program at the Veterans Administration Hospital, 5th Anniversary ed., New York, Veterans Administration Voluntary Service Hospital Advisory Committee, 1955.

TINKER, F.: The Papagos become candy stripers. *Today's Health, 40*:34, 37, 75-76, 1962.

Toledo State Hospital benefits from women's auxiliary. *Ment. Hosp., 3*:6, 1952.

Toy makers. *Auxiliary Leader, 5*:14, 1964.

TRAPP, E.: Help-raising teen-agers. *Recreation Magazine,* December, 1956.

TURNER, J. A.: A volunteer leader's training course. *Recreation Magazine,* September, 1951.

UMBARGER, C. C.; DALSIMER, J. S.; MORRISON, A. P., and BREGGIN, P. R.: *College Students in a Mental Hospital.* New York, Grune, 1962.

VAIL, D. J., and KARLINS, M.: A decade of volunteer services: history and social significance. *Int. J. Soc. Psychiat., 11*:105-109, 1965.

VANDERKLISH, J. E.: Girl Scout hospital aid program: a three-fold asset. *Hosp. Manage., 86*:100, 1958.

Veterans Administration Voluntary Service Special Subcommittee on turnover in volunteer workers in Veterans Administration Field Station. *Veterans Administration Planning Letter No. 56-65*, 1956, pp. 1-27.

Veterans Administration voluntary service. *J. Indiana Med. Ass.*, 49:526, 1956.

Voluntary services. *Baptist Canad. Nurse*, 59:257-259, 1963.

Voluntary services. Unpublished manuscript, Houston, Veterans Administration Hospital.

Voluntary work. *Nurs. Times*, 58:1000, 1962.

Volunteer leaders. *Recreation Magazine*, April, 1952.

Volunteer Participation by Retired and Older Citizens. Report of the 22nd meeting of Veterans Administration Voluntary Service National Advisory Committee, Washington, D. C., Office of the Chief Medical Director, Veterans Administration, April 18-20, 1961.

Volunteer problems discussed. *Ment. Hosp.*, 5:21, 1954.

Volunteer provides companionship therapy. *Ment. Hosp.*, 4:6, 1953.

Volunteer recreation service. *Recreation Magazine*, February, 1954.

Volunteer service to extended at Manteno. *Ment. Hosp.*, 3:6, 1952.

Volunteer success story. *Recreation Magazine*, May, 1950.

Volunteers. *Recreation Magazine*, September, 1951.

Volunteers tutor patients. *Ment. Hosp.*, 7:18, 1956.

Volunteers provide shopping service. *Ment. Hosp.*, 4:15, 1953.

Volunteers in the recreation program. *Recreation Magazine*, May, 1956.

Volunteers can help patients vote. *Hospitals*, 38:66-67, 1964.

WANDERER, Z. W., and STERNLICHT, M.: Psychologists discover the value of volunteers. Psychology student's work with retardates. *Ment. Hosp.*, 15:271-272, 1964.

We all share the burden. *Nurs. Outlook*, 4:75, 1956.

WEINSTEIN, G. J.: Objectives of Veterans Administration day care centers: the volunteers' contributions. *Ment. Hosp.*, 15:216-219, 1964.

WENDEL, L.: Institutional service units: a link between the mentally ill and the world that has forgotten them. *Mod. Hosp.*, 74:69-71, 1950.

What is a do-dad? *Recreation Magazine*, May, 1951.

WHITE, J. V.: County and rural recreation. *Recreation Magazine*, December, 1956.

WHITEFIELD, G. J.: Voluntary assistance in a "long stay" hospital. *The Hospital*, 51:753-754, 1955.

WILFECK: Triggers to action. *Crippled Child*, 34:13-15, 1956.

WILLIAMS, J.: Geriatric citizen as a volunteer. *Recreation of the Ill and Handicapped*, 3:10, 1959.

WILMHURST: Lend a hand, *Nurs. Times*, 58:80-81, 1962.

WOODY, R. J.: *Wisdom to Know.* New York, Funk, 1964.

WYNDHAM, L.: *Candy Stripers.* New York, Messner, 1958.

YONGE, K. A.: Consolidating relationships with the general community. *Ment. Hosp.*, 9:11-14, 1958.

Youth Corps in Montreal hospitals. *Hosp. Admin.*, 4, 1962.

Resource Addresses

The American Legion Auxiliary
777 N. Meridian Street (3rd Floor)
Indianapolis 7, Indiana

The Foundation for Economic Education, Inc.
Irvington-on-Hudson
New York, New York 10533

New Jersey Division of Aging
Trenton 25,
New Jersey

Superintendent of Documents
Government Printing Office
Washington 25, D. C.

Community Council of Greater New York City
345 E. 45th Street
New York, 17, New York

Jewish Community Center
3505 Mayfield Road
Cleveland Heights, Ohio 44118

Adult Education Association of the U. S. A.
1225 Nineteenth Street, N.W.
Washington, D. C. 20036

Association of Junior Leaguers of America, Inc.
The Waldorf-Astoria
New York 22, New York

Public Affairs Pamphlets
22 E. 38th Street
New York 16, New York

Department of Health, Education, & Welfare
National Institute of Mental Health
Bethesda 14, Maryland

Family Service Association of America
44 E. 23rd Street
New York, New York 10010

The National Social Welfare Assembly, Inc.
345 E. 47th Street
New York, New York

Federation of Protestant Welfare Agencies, Inc.
281 Park Avenue, South
New York, New York 10010

United Community Funds and Councils of America
345 E. 46th Street
New York 22, New York

American National Red Cross
17th and D Streets, N.W.
Washington 13, D. C.

National Association for Mental Health
10 Columbus Circle
New York 19, New York

American Hospital Association
840 N. Lake Shore Drive
Chicago 11, Illinois

American Psychiatric Association
1700 18th Street, N.W.
Washington, D. C.

Veterans Administration
Washington, D. C.

Council of Directors of Hospital Volunteers
c/o The Volunteer Bureau
123 W. Madison Street
Chicago 2, Illinois

United Hospital Fund
3 E. 54th Street
New York 22, New York

The National Committee for Mental Hygiene
1790 Broadway
New York, New York

Family Welfare Association of America
122 22nd Street
New York, New York

Mental Health Federation, Inc.
2108 Union Central Building
Cincinnati 2, Ohio

The American Legion
1608 K Street, N.W.
Washington 6, D. C.

American Public Welfare Association
1313 E. 60th Street
Chicago 37, Illinois

Girl Scouts of U. S. A.
830 Third Avenue
New York 22, New York

National Travelers Aid Association
425 Fourth Avenue
New York, New York

National Recreation Association
315 Fourth Avenue
New York 10, New York

Association Press
291 Broadway
New York, New York 10007

Volunteer Community Activities Clearinghouse, Inc.
5507 33rd Street, N.W.
Washington, D. C. 20015

Institute for the Advancement of Volunteer Programs
Center for Continuing Education
Northeastern University
Boston, Massachusetts 02115

Chapter XIV

SIGNIFICANCE OF CONTINUING EDUCATION FOR MAINTENANCE THERAPY*

REUBEN J. MARGOLIN AND BERNARD A. STOTSKY

IT IS MOST fitting that the concluding chapter be devoted to the role of continuing education in maintaining the geriatric patient, for only through this medium can the best in medical care and treatment be provided for the long-term patient. Without continuing education, the physician, nurse, teacher, therapist, psychologist, social worker, aide, and even the maintenance and office workers run the risk of becoming obsolete in the tasks they perform.

By *continuing education* we mean the exposure by formal and informal means of every individual working with the geriatric patient to the latest educational, scientific, and medical developments which sustain his competence in performing professional functions.

The channels for continuing growth and development are quite diverse and range from self-study to formal didactic teaching. Abundant opportunities exist to attend meetings, conferences, institutes, and workshops. Many universities are offering formal training programs in gerontology, geriatrics, and rehabilitation through their basic colleges. In divisions of continuing education a variety of offerings is available on a noncredit basis which reflect the changes occurring in the treatment of the aged. These programs have emerged to meet current needs, and "hot off the press" material constitutes the essence of their curricula.

*Partially supported by grants No. RD -13-10, by V.R.A. and MH 1624-03, by National Institute of Mental Health, U. S. Public Health Service.

In addition to these formal and informal training opportunities, the potential for self-development through personal, systematic effort should not be overlooked. Textbooks, articles in professional journals and popular magazines, as well as radio and television programs bring to our attention new developments in the care and treatment of geriatric patients. Finally, in-service training within the institution and imaginative supervision are powerful vehicles for continuing education.

Why the tremendous emphasis on continuing education at this time? We are living in an era of accelerated social change. History has never before witnessed the rapidity with which social change is occurring today. Education which was once considered terminal (for example, that culminating in AB, MA, or PhD degrees) is now regarded only as prerequisite for the future. The amount of available knowledge is enormous, and we are faced with a crisis not only in accumulating these data, but also in appropriately digesting data for pragmatic application to our daily living.

Terming this modern acceleration a social revolution, as some have, is somewhat misleading; that is only one phase of the development. We must recognize that there is an educational revolution, a scientific revolution, and a medical revolution, all of which have tremendous relevance for both professional and nonprofessional workers in the field of geriatrics.

For example, the educational revolution dramatically emphasizes that most of us are dealing with situations which require training and education not available until recently. In fact, the deficiencies are so prominent at the professional level that an individual who has been in his field for any length of time without continuing his education is not generally considered to be a good prospect for employment or promotion.

Engineers out of school for five years are considered anachronistic because within that time span the flood of new knowledge has changed the complexity of the engineering profession. To cope with these prodigious developments, most companies require that engineers spend at least 20 per cent of their time in continuing education activities. Similarly, the American Academy of General Practitioners, as a requirement for retaining membership in the organization, stipulates that its members must devote at least 20 per cent of their time to continuing education and provide evidence that they are doing so.

Some adults feel threatened by the prospect of being learners for the rest of their lives. Surprisingly, this fear is true of the professional as well as the nonprofessional. The old cliché that "you can't teach an old dog new tricks" is voiced as a rationalization for resisting continuing education. However, the weight of evidence is against this kind of reasoning. Not only can a person learn new things in his later years, but it is essential that he not stop learning. Remaining intellectually alert lays the foundation for a sense of well-being in our later years.

Continuing education is crucial because no professional field can afford to remain static. Alternately in accord and alternately at odds with professionalism is the constant thrust toward advancing frontiers of knowledge and practice. This is especially true in medicine, where changing patterns of illness and medical care are forcing a redefinition of illness and health. The worker in the field of geriatrics cannot avoid the responsibility of sticking to his educational knitting. He may drop a stitch here and there, but with the careful guidance of the adult educator he will not only survive but will prosper amidst the plethora of new knowledge and developments.

The adult educator is aware that the adult learner comes into an educational situation with anxieties and apprehensions. He is skilled in making the learner feel comfortable in what is initially a very stressful situation. Such behavior is not unusual when the adult learner realizes that the knowledge acquired in youth will not be adequate in his mature years and he begins to question his ability to meet the challenge of change. Fortunately, the dearly bought maturity of experience provides a firm foundation for further learning. At the same time, care must be exercised lest these experiences, ideas, attitudes, and interests interfere with modification of professional functions and acquisition of new functions.

Perhaps the most important reason for continuing education is the dilemma of the elder citizen. The statistics regarding the increasing life span are well known and need not be cited. They are a tribute to better control of infectious disease and improved preventive health practices. Let us not forget the disillusionments and distresses of the elderly—the lonely, aimless, at times meaningless lives of the independent and institutionalized aged. Too many persons reach old age with disabling infirmities which for all intents and purposes reduce living to mere survival. The challenge, yet to be met, is to sustain the health, competence, and social status of individuals in the later years of life so that they remain productive and enjoy the benefits of a lifetime of effort.

Continuing education can help to catalyze changes in geriatric care and treatment by developing more effective methods of maintenance therapy and by preparing for the time when medical science converts a maintenance function into a restorative or even a preventive one. Tremendous advances in surgical methods, pharmacology, rehabilitation, and in nutritional management have made it possible even for persons with several chronic diseases to function adequately in coping with the demands of daily living. Throughout this book we have underscored this point. We have provided illustrations whereby the chronic psychiatric patient can be brought to a point of satisfactory remission and then be maintained at this level. Maintenance procedures have been suggested to prevent the crippling deformity of arthritis and the complications of diabetes, hypertension, and other cardiovascular conditions. We have also cautioned that where maintenance therapy has not been initiated or where it has been stopped unwisely, retrogressive changes in function will probably take place.

The knowledge that maintenance measures can be adequate is encouraging, but it is not enough. We must constantly search for more effective methods of maintenance. Reduction of pain, increase in mobility, or improvement in psychological well-being will provide greater guarantees for satisfactory living at any age.

Better methods of maintenance therapy are being developed. The field of pharmacology provides a good example: New drugs are being produced in such great quantities that it is difficult to keep advised of their use in treatment. It has been said that more drugs have been produced in the last ten years than in all medical history. Established standard drugs are being carefully reexamined through research to increase their efficacy and decrease toxicity. Thus, attempts have been made to develop an aspirin which has a measured effect and which is sustained over a longer period of time up to eight hours.

Drugs exercise a maintenance function. They help reduce anxiety, maintain cardiac regularity, improve appetite, increase strength, and maintain regularity of certain bodily functions. Without doubt, drugs have been a boon to the care and treatment of the geriatric patient.

Rehabilitation medicine has also contributed to more effective maintenance therapy. Not too long ago the geriatric patient was not considered an appropriate subject for rehabilitation. Although rehabilitation has always been concerned with the chronically ill, efforts were centered on those patients considered to be medically feasible for employment. However, innovations and new approaches in medicine and the social sciences have changed the prevailing climate of opinion. For example, developments in cardiology such as the pace-maker, open-heart surgery, heart-monitoring devices, and judicious use of exercise result in an increased number of patients considered good candidates for rehabilitation.

Inherent in the rehabilitation process is the concept of maintenance. Rehabilitation is ineffective unless the patient learns to maintain himself, capitalizing on abilities to overcome disabilities.

As a corollary to this increased activity in rehabilitation, the aging patient has been recognized as an acceptable candidate for rehabilitation. Today we often read about the successful rehabilitation, even to the point of reemployment, of patients.

In fact, the senior author had the pleasure of working with a patient (discussed in Chapter II) who returned to work at the age of sixty-five after twenty years of hospitalization and continued to work until he was eighty years old. During this period the physician, the counseling psychologist, the social worker, the rehabilitation nurse, the employer, the foster mother, and members of his real family all contributed significantly to maintaining this patient in a state of well-being, despite the fact that he was afflicted with several diseases. In the case of each person involved, continuing education was important. The physician experimented with a variety of new drugs and approaches to medical care, all of which required his keeping abreast of recent medical thinking. This same situation applied to all the other members involved. The chief responsibilities of the social worker and the counseling psychologist were to discover the patient's potential for successful rehabilitation and to help provide the means for achieving such a result.

Continuing education is important in an era of great medical achievements, because with each new medical development, new methods for education and training will be necessary. Since World War II, many new health careers have emerged. With renewed education comes the need for comparable changes in attitudes as the outlook for successful treatment improves.

A primary objective of medical research is to restore normal functioning. Most advances make a contribution to the area of maintenance therapy. The new field of space medicine has introduced exciting new ideas which are potentially applicable to rehabilitation. Electronics also promises to have significant ramifications in teaching speech to the congenitally deaf and the aphasic patient. Neurosensory studies are being carried out which concern the blind and the deaf. Even more remarkable is the possibility that the deaf may communicate over the telephone by means of electronic attachments. Similarly, a new invention announced by the New York Telephone Company enables totally paralyzed persons to use the phone with the aid of a headset and chin-level microswitch. It is hoped that mobility of the nonambulatory patient will also be increased through the use of electronics. Servomechanisms are now being used in experiments to energize paralyzed muscles. One of the most inspiring creations is an electronically powered wheelchair which goes up and down stairs. These and many other developments are opening up new possibilities for a more productive, more active life for the handicapped.

Another development worthy of note is the advance in computer technology. The use of computers in diagnosis of medical conditions and in assisting social workers and rehabilitation counselors with intake procedures is now being explored.

Operant conditioning is being used to treat autistic children and severe schizophrenics. Programmed instruction has already proven valuable in teaching mentally retarded patients and those with cerebral palsy as well as hemiplegic patients. Computers are also being used in administration to effect improvements in management of hospitals and other health agencies through systems analysis and more efficient data-processing procedures. All these innovations enhance the process of maintenance therapy.

Legislative and societal pressures may also enhance comprehensive maintenance therapy through development of more effective systems of medical care and research. It is too early to assess the impact of Medicare or that of the regional heart, stroke, and cancer centers, but it is already evident that hospital services and extended care facilities are being heavily utilized for the treatment of geriatric patients. The extended care facility, neither a nursing home nor a convalescent hospital, has been created in response to the requirements of the Medicare Act (Public Law 89-97) for up to one hundred days of skilled nursing care, rehabilitation, casework, and medical care during the period after hospitalization. Prominent among the requirements is the presence of rehabilitative activities to maintain the patient at a satisfactory level. As a result of Medicare, new kinds of facilities for geriatric care will appear on the American scene.

Perhaps the legislation will spur the development of communities for the older citizen based around the extended care facility, complexes containing a variety of transitional facilities including general hospitals, mental hospitals with day care and night care plans, nursing homes, homes for the aged, outpatient clinics, halfway houses, special housing for the elderly, community recreational centers, and shopping centers.

Finally, the impact of the antipoverty program must be considered. It has forced the nation to confront the enormous health and social problems arising from inadequate living situations. Such environments breed ignorance and distorted values within the family structure and result in poor hygiene and neglect of medical conditions. Community health centers have been established to explore new techniques for the treatment and health education of the poor. As a result, all individuals, including the aged, in the "poverty culture" are being given the opportunity to function at a higher maintenance level.

The basic goal of continuing education is to maintain proficient professional performance in treatment of the aged through exposure to the latest developments in health, education, and welfare. Emphasis must be placed on attitudes as well as on education and training. Bernard Baruch once said, "There is no such thing as a human scrap heap." Horace Mann exhorted, "Be afraid to die unless you achieve some victory for humanity." These two statements eloquently underscore the significance of continuing education for maintenance therapy.

NAME INDEX

Alexander, Marie M., 109
Allen, J., 53, 70
Anderson, Thomas P., M.D., 64-65
Arffa, Marvin S., 248

Barry, J. R., 95, 107
Baxt, R., 44, 45, 47
Barron, F., 6, 26
Baruch, Bernard, 283
Bechill, William D., 236
Beck, J. C., 250, 257
Bell, Benjamin, 187
Best, E. E., 40, 47
Bonnet, Dr., 231
Bortz, Dr. Edward Leroy, 18, 57, 71
Brooke, C. K., 30, 45
Brown, Dr. J. Harold, 182, 186
Bunim, Joseph, M. D., 174-175, 186

Caplan, Gerald, 74
Calabro, 176, 186
Chasen, William H., 174
Costello, J. P., Jr., 28, 45
Cragg, Charles I., 21, 27
Cureton, Thomas K., Jr., Ph.D., 18, 27, 57, 59, 60, 71

Davis, J. E., 35, 46
Day, Dr. P. L.
Dill, D. B., 50, 70

Engerbretson, L., 67, 72

Fox, J., 56, 71

Galineau, V., 250, 257
Gerontinos, E. M., 51, 70
Goldin, George J., 95, 107
Goldner, Dr. J. Leonard, 184 186
Goldstein, M. S., 67, 72
Graber, J. B., 213, 226
Granning, Dr. Harold M., 234
Guild, W. R., 56, 71

Hadley, William B., 158
Harter, 185, 186
Hellerstein, Dr. Herman K., 18, 57, 59, 71
Hess, Arthur E., 229-230, 232
Honigfeld, G., 142, 151
Hulicka, 39, 47
Hunt, James C., 228
Hurwitz, F. L., 23

Jokl, E., 56, 71

Kantor, D., 250, 257
Kendall, 175, 186
Keyes, Ancel, 65, 70
Knudson, Dr. A. B. C., 15, 27, 45, 47
Krauss, H., 52, 70
Krauss, T., 31, 46

Le Guin, K. W., 33, 46
Leiberman, J. M., 38, 47

285

SUBJECT INDEX

A

ACTH, 183, 185
Activity programs, ix, 49, 154
Adhesions, 9
Adjustment difficulties, 132-135
Adrenocorticotropic hormone therapy, 175, 185-186
Administration on Aging, 83-84, 236, 247
Age Center, 226
Agitation, 147, 148, 150
Aid to the Permanently and Totally Disabled, 80
Albert Einstein Medical Center, Philadelphia, 182
Alcoholism, 133, 148
Allopurinal, 178
Ambulation, 48, 52, 66
American Academy of General Practitioners, 277-278
American Cancer Society, 37, 93, 217
American College of Physicians, 219
American College of Radiologists, 231
American College of Surgeons, 219,
American Congress of Physical Medicine and Rehabilitation, 62, 63
American Dental Association, 244
American Diabetes Association, 162
American Dietetic Association, 162
American Heart Association, 56, 71, 217
American Hospital Association, 217
American Medical Association, 217, 219, 244
American Nurses' Association, 217
American Osteopathic Association, 244
American Public Health Association, 217
Amitriptyline, 149-150
Amputation, 52, 159, 169-170
Ankylosing spondylitis, 176-177, 179
Anesthesiology, 151, 230-231

Antidepressant drugs, 150
Antipoverty program, 282
Anturin, 178
Anxiety, 178
Arteries, 5, 188, 189
Arthritis, 5, 65
    patients, 174-186
Arthritis Foundation, 178
Atrophy, 9, 51
Attitudes, 7, 76-77
Autistic patients, 282

B

Backache, 52-53
Barbiturates, 144, 146, 150-151, 152
Bed exercises, 48, 52
    see also, Exercises
Bed rest, 52, 66
Beebe loupe, 190
Behavior problems, 132-135
Benemid, 178, 180
Benztropine mesylate, 147
Bethany Methodist Home and Hospital, 246
Bingham Association Fund, 219
Biperidene, 147
Blood Dyscrasias, 180
Blood pressure, 59
Blue Cross-Blue Shield, 218, 219, 232
Boston Dispensary Program, 222
Brain syndromes, 136
British antileucite, 175
Bureau of Family Services, 203
Bureau of Medical Services, 203, 204
Bureau of State Services, 203, 204
Bursitis, 183
Butazone, 180

C

Calcium, 112
Calories, 114

287